DUKAN DIET 2024

120 Recipes The Complete Guide to the Four Phases, A Modern Approach and the Secret to losing weight Without Giving up

TERY LONG

DISCLAIMER

Please note that the content of this book is based on personal experience and various sources of information. This book aims to provide useful and informative material on the topics covered in the publication. It is sold with the understanding that the author and publisher are not engaged in rendering any personal medical, health care, or other professional services in the book. The reader should consult his or her physician, health care provider, or other competent professional before adopting any suggestions in this book or drawing any conclusions. The author and publisher expressly disclaim any responsibility for any liability, loss, or risk, personal or otherwise, arising, directly or indirectly, from the use and application of any contents of this book.

NOTE

In the context of this book, when we refer to "a cup" as a unit of measurement for ingredients, we mean using a standard kitchen cup with a capacity of approximately 2 milliliters. It is essential to use a measuring cup to get the right quantities of ingredients. If you don't have a measuring cup, you can use a graduated measuring cup, making sure to correctly correspond to the proportions indicated. Here are some examples 1 Cup of flour 100 gr. 1 cup of rice 200 gr. 1 Cup of Quinoa 200 g, It is recommended to level the dry ingredients in the cup using a spatula or the blade of a knife to obtain an accurate measurement. For liquid ingredients it is recommended to fill the cup to the brim without squeezing or leaving gaps.

RECIPES FOR BREAKFAST

RECIPES APPETIZERS

ATTACK PHASE

CRUISE PHASE

83 CHICKEN SALAD WITH GRILLED VEGETABLES

85 SMOKED SALMON MOUSSE WITH GREEK YOGURT

87 BEET CARPACCIO WITH RICOTTA

89 SHRIMP AND COURGETTE SKEWERS

91 STUFFED EGGS WITH TUNA AND GREEK YOGURT

93 SEAFOOD SALAD WITH VEGETABLES

95 SALMON CARPACCIO WITH YOGURT AND CHIVE SAUCE

97 COURGETTE FRITTERS WITH MINT AND LEMON

99 PEPPER ROLLS WITH TUNA AND BLACK OLIVES

CONSOLIDATION PHASE

101 QUINOA SALAD WITH GRILLED VEGETABLES AND FETA

103 WHOLE WHOLE BRUSCHETTAS WITH TOMATOES AND FRESH BASIL

105 CAPRESE WITH TOMATO, LIGHT MOZZARELLA AND BASIL

107 WHOLE BREAD CANAPES WITH AVOCADO AND SMOKED SALMON

109 BUCKWHEAT FRITTERS WITH COURGETTES AND PARMESAN

111 LENTIL SALAD WITH ROASTED PEPPERS AND TUNA

113 GRILLED AUBERGINES ROLLS WITH COOKED HAM AND LIGHT CHEESE

115 WHOLE BREAD CROUTTONS WITH RICOTTA CREAM AND DRIED TOMATOES

117 CHICKEN SALAD WITH MANGO, AVOCADO AND SUNFLOWER SEEDS

STABILIZATION PHASE

119 GREEK SALAD WITH TOMATOES, CUCUMBERS, PEPPERS, OLIVES AND FETA

121 AVOCADO CARPACCIO WITH PRAWNS AND MANGO

123 WHOLE WHOLE BRUSCHETTE WITH TOMATOES, BASIL AND BUFFALO MOZZARELLA

RECIPES FIRST DISHES

ATTACK PHASE

CRUISE PHASE

CONSOLIDATION PHASE

STABILIZATION PHASE

RECIPES SECOND DISHES

ATTACK PHASE

220 ASPARAGUS AND MUSHROOM OMELETTES

222 STEAMED SALMON WITH LEMON SAUCE AND HERBS

224 GRILLED BEEF FILLET WITH ROASTED TOMATOES

226 GRILLED SWORDFISH WITH SPINACH SIDE SIDE

228 TUNA SALAD WITH TOMATOES AND CUCUMBERS

230 BAKED COD FILLET WITH TOMATOES AND OREGANO

CRUISE PHASE

232 CHICKEN CURRY WITH GRILLED VEGETABLES

234 GRILLED SALMON WITH CITRUS SAUCE

236 BEEF STEAK WITH PEPPERS AND ONIONS

238 CHICKEN BREAST STUFFED WITH SPINACH AND SKINNY CHEESE

CONSOLIDATION PHASE

263 VEGETABLE OMELETE WITH LIGHT CHEESE

STABILIZATION PHASE

265 SEA SEABASS WITH SEASONAL VEGETABLES

267 CHICKEN SCALOPPINE WITH MUSHROOMS WITH MASHED POTATOES

270 TURKEY BURGER WITH WHEEL BREAD AND GRILLED VEGETABLES

272 SALMON FILLET IN PISTACHIO CRUST WITH WHOLE WHOLE COUSCOUS

274 BEEF STEAK WITH GRILLED PEPPERS

276 AUBERGINES ROLLS WITH VEGETABLES AND LIGHT CHEESE

278 SLICED BEEF WITH MIXED SALAD AND SEASONED TOMATOES

280 SWORDFISH WITH LEMON WITH BULGUR AND VEGETABLES

SIDE DISH RECIPES

ATTACK PHASE

283 CUCUMBERS AND TOMATO SALAD WITH APPLE VINEGAR AND AROMATIC HERBS

285 GRILLED ASPARAGUS WITH OLIVE OIL AND BLACK PEPPER

287 SAUTEED CHAMPIGNON MUSHROOMS WITH GARLIC AND PARSLEY

CRUISE PHASE

289 GRILLED COURGETTES WITH PEPPERS AND ONIONS

291 BAKED AUBERGINES WITH TOMATO AND BASIL SAUCE

293 MIXED SALAD WITH CHICORY, LETTUCE, ROCKET AND GRATED CARROTS

CONSOLIDATION PHASE

295 COLD QUINOA WITH PEPPERS, TOMATOES AND BLACK OLIVES

297 BAKED SWEET POTATOES WITH ROSEMARY AND GARLIC

299 COURGETTE FLAN WITH RICOTTA AND EGGS

STABILIZATION PHASE

301 WHOLE WHOLE COUSCOUS WITH GRILLED VEGETABLES AND FRESH MINT

303 BAKED POTATOES WITH ROSEMARY AND GARLIC

305 MIXED VEGETABLE OMELETTE WITH SPINACH, TOMATOES AND COURGETTES

INTRODUCTION DUKAN DIET

The Dukan Diet is a high-protein diet, which promotes rapid weight loss and the elimination of excess kilos. Welcome to the 2024 Dukan Diet, an updated and comprehensive guide to achieving your weight loss and health goals through a scientifically proven and sustainable approach. Founded by Dr. Pierre Dukan in 1972, the Dukan Diet has gained popularity around the world for its effectiveness in promoting weight loss without sacrificing health or food satisfaction. Over the years, the Dukan Diet has been the subject of continuous research and development, adapting to the needs and latest scientific discoveries in the field of nutrition and health. In this 2024 edition, we will explore the fundamental principles of the Dukan Diet, its four distinctive phases, and strategies for long-term success.

Through the balance between lean proteins, vegetables, and the gradual replenishment of other foods, the Dukan Diet not only promotes weight loss, but also the building of healthy and sustainable eating habits. Each phase of the program is designed to offer a gradual, controlled progression, allowing your body to adapt and achieve lasting results. In this book, we will explore every aspect of the 2024 Dukan Diet in detail, providing practical advice, tips for success and testimonials from those who have embraced this approach and transformed their lives. With the Dukan Diet, you learn to make smart choices, enjoy delicious, nutritious meals, and achieve optimal fitness without compromising your health. We hope this book will be a valuable resource for those looking to transform their bodies and lives through the Dukan Diet.

HISTORY AND PHILOSOPHY OF THE DUKAN DIET

The Dukan Diet is a high-protein, low-carb diet, created by French nutritionist Dr. Pierre Dukan. Its philosophy is based on the idea that consuming a high amount of protein and reducing carbohydrates can promote weight loss quickly and sustainably. Origins of the Dukan Diet The Dukan Diet has its roots in the 1970s, when Dr. Pierre Dukan was working as a general practitioner in France. One day, an overweight patient expressed the desire to lose weight without having to give up meat. This led Dukan to consider the idea of a diet that allowed the consumption of protein foods, while limiting carbohydrates and fats. After successfully testing his approach on several patients. The Dukan Diet is one of the best known diets in the world. mb3ìPhilosophy of the Dukan Diet The philosophy of the Dukan Diet is based on some key principles:

1. High Protein Consumption: Proteins are at the center of the diet, as they require more energy to digest and metabolize than carbohydrates or fats. This process, called the thermogenic effect, can help you burn more calories. Additionally, protein helps maintain muscle mass during weight loss and promotes greater satiety. 2. Reduction of Carbohydrates and Fats: The diet drastically reduces the intake of carbohydrates and fats, pushing the body to use fat reserves as its main source of energy. This state, known as ketosis, can accelerate weight loss. 3. Progressive Phases: The Dukan Diet is divided into four phases (Attack, Cruise, Consolidation and Stabilization), each of which has specific objectives and guidelines. This gradual approach helps people lose weight safely and maintain long-term results. 4. Long-Term Maintenance: Once the ideal weight has been reached, the diet includes a stabilization phase that allows a gradual return to a more balanced diet, while maintaining some rules to prevent weight

regain. 5. Simplicity and Structure: The Dukan Diet provides a structured, easy-to-follow eating plan, with a clear list of permitted and prohibited foods. This can help reduce uncertainty and temptation, making it easier to stick to the diet. In summary, the Dukan Diet combines a scientific approach to nutrition with a clear, workable structure, making it a popular choice for those looking to lose weight and keep it off over time. However, it is important to remember that each diet has its pros and cons and may not be suitable for everyone.

WHY CHOOSE THE DUKAN DIET

The Dukan Diet has been chosen by millions of people around the world for several reasons. Here are some of the main reasons why many decide to follow this diet: 1. Rapid and Effective Weight Loss Visible Results in a Short Time: The initial "Attack" phase of the Dukan Diet is designed to stimulate rapid weight loss, motivating whoever follows her to continue. Carbohydrate restriction and high protein consumption cause the body to burn fat more efficiently. Motivational Effect: Rapid initial results can be very motivating, especially for those who need to see concrete progress to stay engaged. 2. Satiety and Appetite Reduction High Protein Consumption: Proteins are macronutrients known to promote prolonged satiety. By consuming foods rich in proteins, you can reduce the feeling of hunger and cravings, making it easier to comply with the rules of the diet. Reduce Sugar Cravings: Limiting carbohydrates, especially refined carbohydrates, helps stabilize blood sugar levels, reducing cravings for sweet foods and simple carbohydrates. 3. Clear Structure and Simplicity Well-Defined Phases: The Dukan Diet is divided into four phases (Attack, Cruise, Consolidation and Stabilization), each with precise guidelines. This structure helps you know exactly what to eat at each stage, reducing uncertainty and making it easier to stick to the diet. Allowed Food List: Provides a detailed list of allowed foods, making meal planning and shopping easier. 4. Long-Term Maintenance Stabilization Phase: Once the desired weight has been reached, the Dukan Diet introduces a maintenance phase that allows a gradual return to a more balanced diet, with clear rules to prevent weight regain. Flexibility: The phase of Stabilization allows for greater dietary freedom, making the diet sustainable in the long term without completely giving up favorite foods. 5. Adaptability and Variety Adaptable to Different Needs: The Dukan Diet can be customized to suit various dietary needs, including those of vegetarians and people with food intolerances. Wide Choice of Foods: Although limited in some categories, the diet offers a wide range of protein-rich foods, including lean meats, fish, eggs, low-fat dairy products and legumes. 6. Nutrition Education Awareness of Food Choices: Following the Dukan Diet can increase awareness of one's food choices and macronutrients, helping people make more informed choices even after completing the program. In summary, the Dukan Diet offers a combination of rapid weight loss, satiety, structure and long-term sustainability, making it an attractive choice for many people.

THE FOUR PHASES OF THE DUKAN DIET

The Dukan Diet is structured into four distinct phases, each with specific goals and dietary guidelines. This gradual approach is designed to promote rapid weight loss and long-term stabilization.1. Attack Phase Duration: From 1 to 7 days, depending on the weight to be lost. Objective: Promote rapid initial weight loss to motivate those following the diet. Allowed foods: Pure proteins (PP): lean meat (chicken, turkey, beef), fish, seafood, eggs, tofu, low-fat dairy products (yogurt, low-fat cheese), vegetable proteins. Drinks: water, tea, coffee without sugar. Seasonings: herbs, spices, vinegar, lemon juice (in limited quantities), mustard, salt and pepper (in moderation). Characteristics: This phase allows you to quickly lose weight thanks to the high protein intake and the almost total elimination of carbohydrates and fats. Protein helps maintain muscle mass and promote the feeling of satiety. 2. Cruise Phase Duration: Until reaching ideal weight. Goal: Continue gradual and steady weight loss. Allowed foods: Alternation of Pure Protein (PP) days and Protein and Vegetable (PV) days. Pure proteins as in the Attack phase. Low-starch vegetables: tomatoes, spinach, broccoli, cabbage, cucumbers, peppers, zucchini, mushrooms, asparagus, green beans, etc. Others: a teaspoon of oat bran per day to aid digestion and increase satiety. Characteristics: During this phase, protein-only days alternate with days in which vegetables are added, promoting constant weight loss. It is important to maintain protein intake to preserve muscle mass. 3. Consolidation Phase Duration: 10 days for every kilo lost during the previous phases. Objective: Prevent regaining lost weight and begin gradually reintroducing other foods into your diet. Food

Allowed: All foods from the previous phases. Gradual introduction of fruit (1 serving per day, excluding bananas, grapes and cherries), wholemeal bread (2 slices per day), cheese (40g per day), and limited portions of carbohydrates (2 servings per week). One "gala" meal per week: any food is allowed, but in moderation and without encores. Characteristics: This phase is crucial to stabilize the new weight. Gradually introducing previously excluded foods helps reintroduce a more balanced and sustainable diet. 4. Stabilization Phase Duration: Indeterminate (for life). Goal: Maintain the weight achieved in the long term. Guidelines: Continue to follow the principles of the Consolidation Phase, but with greater flexibility. One day a week of Pure Protein (usually Thursdays). Continue to maintain regular physical activity. Characteristics: This phase involves maintaining the healthy eating habits acquired during the diet.

NUTRITIONAL PRINCIPLES OF THE DUKAN DIET

The Dukan Diet is based on some fundamental principles that aim to promote weight loss, maintain muscle mass and improve overall health. Here are the main nutritional concepts of the diet: 1. High Protein Consumption Benefits of Proteins: Satiety: Proteins take longer to digest than carbohydrates and fats, which helps maintain the feeling of satiety longer. This can reduce overall calorie consumption, making weight loss easier. Maintaining Muscle Mass: During weight loss, it is important to preserve muscle mass to maintain an active metabolism. Protein provides the amino acids needed to build and repair muscles. Thermogenic Effect: Digestion of proteins requires more energy, increasing the body's calorie expenditure.

This thermogenic effect can contribute to greater weight loss. Sources of Protein: Lean meat, fish, eggs, low-fat dairy products, plant proteins such as tofu and legumes. 2. Reducing Carbohydrates Reasons for Reducing Carbs: Ketonemia: By drastically reducing your carbohydrate intake, the body enters a state called ketosis, in which it uses fat as its main source of energy. Stabilizing Blood Sugar Levels: A low carbohydrate intake helps avoid blood sugar spikes and dips, reducing cravings for sugary foods and promoting steadier energy. Allowed Carbohydrates: During the initial stages of the diet, carbohydrates are limited almost exclusively to those found in vegetables. In later stages, complex carbohydrates such as wholemeal bread, wholemeal pasta and brown rice can be reintroduced in a controlled manner. 3. Fat Reduction Why Limit Fat: Caloric Density: Fat is the macronutrient with

The higher calorie density (9 calories per gram), so reducing your consumption can help control your total calorie intake. Choosing Healthy Fats: Although the diet limits fat intake, it promotes consumption of healthy fats found in fatty fish (such as salmon and tuna), avocados and vegetable oils in small amounts. 4. Hydration and Importance of Water Role of Hydration: Digestion and Metabolism: Drinking water is essential for the proper functioning of the metabolism and to aid digestion, especially with high protein consumption. Detoxification: Water helps flush toxins from the body and prevent constipation, a possible side effect of a high-protein diet. Satiety: Drinking water before meals can help reduce appetite and avoid calorie overload. 5. Benefits of Oat Bran:

Source of Fibre: Oat bran is rich in soluble fibre, which helps regulate intestinal transit and improve digestion. Satiety: Soluble fiber forms a gel-like substance in the stomach, which can increase feelings of fullness. Blood Sugar Control: Fiber can help control blood sugar levels by reducing the absorption of carbohydrates. 6. Physical Activity Incorporation of Exercise: Weight Loss Support: Regular physical activity helps burn calories, maintain muscle mass and improve cardiovascular health. Diet Recommended: The Dukan Diet encourages exercise, such as daily walks, to support weight loss and improve overall well-being. These nutritional principles are the basis of the Dukan Diet and aim to promote effective and sustainable weight loss.

BENEFITS OF THE DUKAN DIET

The Dukan Diet is popular for a number of benefits it offers to those who follow it. Here are some of the main benefits: 1. Quick and Effective Weight Loss One of the main reasons why many people choose the Dukan Diet is the promise of rapid weight loss. The initial "Attack" phase is designed to promote rapid reduction in body weight, which can be very motivating for those starting the diet. This result is achieved through a drastic reduction in carbohydrates and a high consumption of proteins, which promote ketosis and fat burning. 2. Increased Satiety and Reduced Appetite High protein consumption is a key feature of the Dukan Diet. Protein is known to be more satiating than carbohydrates and fats, which can help reduce your overall calorie intake. This effect is due to the fact that proteins take longer to digest and increase the production of satiety hormones, such as peptide YY and GLP1. 3. Preservation of Muscle Mass During weight loss, one of the main risks is the loss of muscle mass. The Dukan Diet, with its high protein intake, helps preserve lean mass while losing fat. This is especially important because muscles play a crucial role in maintaining basal metabolic rate. 4. Regulation of Blood Sugar Levels Reducing carbohydrates in the diet can help stabilize blood sugar levels, reducing the risk of blood sugar spikes and drops. This may be especially beneficial for people with prediabetes or type 2 diabetes, as it helps improve insulin sensitivity. 5. Structure and Ease of Following the Diet The Dukan Diet is structured into four well-defined phases, each with clear guidelines on which foods are allowed.

This framework helps people know exactly what they can eat at each stage, reducing uncertainty and making it easier to stick to the diet. Additionally, permitted food lists make meal planning and shopping easier. 6. Long-Term Maintenance The final phase of the diet, "Stabilization," is designed to help people maintain lost weight long-term. This phase introduces greater dietary flexibility and includes one day of pure protein per week to maintain results. This balanced approach makes the diet more sustainable in the long run than many other crash diets. 7. Reducing Cholesterol and Improving Cardiovascular Health Some studies have suggested that a diet high in protein and low in carbohydrates can help reduce levels of LDL cholesterol (the "bad cholesterol") and improve the lipid profile.

This can have positive effects on cardiovascular health, reducing the risk of heart disease. 8. Nutrition Education Following the Dukan Diet can increase awareness of your food choices and macronutrients. This can lead to a greater understanding of the foods you consume and their health implications, promoting healthier eating habits even after you quit the diet. It is important to note that, as with any diet, the Dukan Diet may not be suitable for everyone and may present some risks, especially if followed for long periods or without medical supervision. Therefore, it is advisable to consult a health professional before starting this or any other diet

DUKAN RECIPES: EXAMPLES OF DISHES FOR EACH PHASE OF THE DIET

Attack phase (pure protein):

Breakfast:

Scrambled eggs with cooked ham

0% Greek yogurt with chia seeds

Light cream cheese

Lunch:

Baked salmon with herbs

Grilled chicken with a green salad

Steamed mussels

Dinner:

Roasted turkey steak

Sautéed shrimp with vegetables

Steamed cod, ginger sauce

Cruise phase (protein + vegetables):

Breakfast:

Dukan biscuits with ham and cheese

Spinach omelette

0% Greek yogurt with low-glycemic fruit (such as kiwi or melon)

Lunch:

Chicken salad with avocado and cherry tomatoes

Baked salmon with grilled vegetables, Lentil soup

Dinner:

Lean meatballs in tomato sauce

Steamed salmon with yogurt sauce, Cuttlefish with potatoes

Consolidation phase:

Breakfast:

Dukan biscuits with light jam

0% Greek yogurt with dried fruit

Vegetable omelette

Lunch:

Tuna salad with potatoes

Chicken curry and basmati rice

Fish soup

Dinner:

Roast beef with vegetables

Baked salmon with sweet potatoes

Light quiche

Stabilization phase:

One day a week of pure protein: you can repeat the menus from the attack phase. Free days: You can gradually introduce other foods in moderation and consider the quantities.

CONCLUSION AND FUTURE OF THE DUKAN DIET

The Dukan Diet has proven to be an effective strategy for weight loss and long-term maintenance, thanks to its clear structure and focus on protein. Through the four well-defined phases, it offers a path that not only promotes rapid weight loss but also the stabilization and maintenance of the weight achieved. With the "Dukan Diet 2024", you have a new and modernized approach that integrates the latest nutritional discoveries and adapts to different dietary needs. The Future of the Dukan Diet Looking ahead, the Dukan Diet will continue to evolve to meet the needs of an ever-changing world.

Emerging food trends, such as a focus on sustainability and the inclusion of plant-based protein alternatives, will be increasingly integrated into this diet. Nutritional research will continue to refine and adapt the guidelines, ensuring that the Dukan Diet remains relevant and safe for all. Additionally, the growing availability of digital resources, food tracking apps and online communities will provide even greater support to dieters, offering practical tools to maintain motivation and track progress. Your Participation Matters Thank you for embarking on this journey with "Dukan Diet 2024". I hope that the book has been helpful to you and that you have found inspiration and guidance to achieve your health goals.

RECIPES
FOR BREAKFAST

ATTACK PHASE

PROTEIN PANCAKES WITH OAT BRAN

Preparation time: 10 minutes

Cooking time: 2-3 minutes per pancake

Doses for 1 person: 2-3 pancakes

Ingredients:

50 g of oat bran

2 egg whites

1 tablespoon protein powder (optional)

1/2 ripe banana

1 teaspoon baking powder

1 pinch of salt

Coconut oil or cooking spray to grease the pan

Fresh fruit and maple syrup (optional) for garnish

Preparation

In a bowl, blend the banana until puree. Add the oat bran, egg whites, protein powder, baking powder and salt. Mix well until you obtain a homogeneous mixture. Heat a non-stick pan over medium heat and lightly grease it. Pour a ladle of mixture for each pancake and cook for 2-3 minutes per side, or until golden brown. Serve warm with fresh fruit and maple syrup, if desired.

Estimated nutritional values (per serving):

Calories: 250-300 kcal

Protein: 25-30g

Carbohydrates: 25-30g

Fat: 5-10g

EGG WHITE AND VEGETABLE OMELETTE

Preparation time: 15 minutes

Cooking time: 15-20 minutes

Doses for 1 person: 1 portion

Ingredients:

4 egg whites

1/2 onion chopped

1/2 chopped pepper

1/4 of a courgette cut into julienne strips

20g grated cheese (optional)

Salt and Pepper To Taste

Extra virgin olive oil

Preparation

In a non-stick pan, heat a drizzle of oil and fry the onion, pepper and courgette until tender. In a bowl, beat the egg whites with a fork until frothy. Add the salt and pepper. Pour the vegetables into the bowl with the egg whites and mix gently. Transfer the mixture to the pan and cook over medium-low heat for 5-7 minutes, or until the omelette is set on the bottom. Sprinkle with the grated cheese and cook under the oven grill for a few minutes, or until the cheese is melted and golden.

Estimated nutritional values (per serving):

Calories: 150-200 kcal

Protein: 20-25g

Carbohydrates: 5-10g

Fat: 5-10g

GREEK YOGURT WITH CHIA SEEDS AND BERRIES

Preparation time: 5 minutes

Cooking time: Not necessary

Doses for 1 person: 1 portion

Ingredients:

1 jar of Greek yogurt (natural or fruit)

1 tablespoon chia seeds

Mixed berries (blueberries, raspberries, blackberries)

Fresh fruit to taste (banana, kiwi, mango)

Honey or maple syrup (optional)

Preparation

Pour the Greek yogurt into a jar or bowl. Add the chia seeds and mix well. Cover the jar and let it rest in the refrigerator for at least 30 minutes, or overnight, for the chia seeds to swell. Before serving, add the wild berries and fresh fruit cut into pieces. If desired, sweeten with honey or maple syrup.

Estimated nutritional values (per serving):

Calories: 150-200 kcal

Protein: 15-20g

Carbohydrates: 15-20g

Fat: 5-10g

CRUISE PHASE

PROTEIN COCOA MUFFINS

Preparation time: 20 minutes

Cooking time: 20-25 minutes

Doses for 6 muffins

Ingredients:

100g of oatmeal

30g of cocoa protein powder

2 whole eggs

1 ripe banana

40ml of milk (vegetable or cow's milk)

30ml of coconut oil

1 teaspoon baking powder

1 pinch of salt

Chopped dark chocolate

(optional) to decorate

Preparation

Preheat the oven to 180°C. In a bowl, mash the banana with a fork. Add eggs, coconut oil, milk, oat flour, protein powder, baking powder, and salt. Mix well until you obtain a homogeneous mixture. If desired, add chopped dark chocolate. Divide the mixture into 6 muffin molds lined with baking paper. Bake for 20-25 minutes, or until golden brown.

Let cool before serving.

Estimated nutritional values (per muffin):

Calories: 150-200 kcal

Protein: 15-20g

Carbohydrates: 20-25g

Fat: 5-10g

BRAN CREPES WITH RICOTTA AND CINNAMON

Preparation time: 20 minutes

Cooking time: 2-3 minutes for crepes

Doses for 6 crepes

Ingredients:

100g of oat bran

2 whole eggs

250 ml of milk (vegetable or cow's milk)

1 pinch of salt

1 teaspoon ground cinnamon

Coconut oil or cooking spray to grease the pan

Fresh ricotta

Fresh mint (optional) for garnish

Preparation

In a blender, blend the oat bran until it becomes a fine flour. In a bowl, beat the eggs with the milk, salt and cinnamon. Add the bran flour and mix well until you obtain a smooth mixture without lumps. Heat a non-stick pan over medium heat and lightly grease it. Pour a ladle of mixture for each crepe and cook for 2-3 minutes per side, or until golden. Fill the crepes with ricotta and garnish with a few fresh mint leaves.

Estimated nutritional values (per serving):

Calories: 150-200 kcal

Protein: 10-15g

Carbohydrates: 20-25g

Fat: 5-10g

OAT BRAN AND ALMOND MILK PORRIDGE

Preparation time: 5 minutes

Cooking time: 5 minutes

Doses for 1 person

Ingredients:

50g of oat bran

250ml of almond milk

1 sliced banana

1 tablespoon chia seeds

Dried fruit to taste (almonds, walnuts)

Ground cinnamon to taste

Preparation

In a saucepan, pour the oat bran and almond milk. Bring to the boil, then lower the heat and leave to cook for about 5 minutes, stirring occasionally, until you obtain a creamy consistency. Pour the porridge into a bowl and add the sliced banana, chia seeds, dried fruit and cinnamon. Mix well and serve immediately.

Estimated nutritional values (per serving):

Calories: 250-300 kcal

Protein: 10-15g

Carbohydrates: 30-35g

Fat: 5-10g

CONSOLIDATION PHASE
PROTEIN OMELETTE

Preparation time: 5 minutes

Cooking time: 5-7 minutes

Doses: 1 person

Ingredients:

2 eggs

20g of lean hard cheese

(like Grana Padano) grated

20g of fresh spinach

Salt and Pepper To Taste

Preparation

Beat the eggs in a bowl, add the grated cheese, finely chopped spinach, salt and pepper. Heat a non-stick pan with a drizzle of oil and pour the mixture. Cook the omelette over medium heat, lifting the edges with a spatula to allow the egg to thicken inside as well. Serve hot.

Estimated nutritional values (per serving):

Calories: 150-200 kcal

Protein: 20-25g

Carbohydrates: 2-3g

Fat: 8-10g

SMOKED SALMON WITH FRESH CHEESE

Preparation time: 5 minutes

Cooking time: Not necessary

Doses: 1 person

Ingredients:

80g of smoked salmon

50g of fresh spreadable cheese

(like Philadelphia)

1 slice of wholemeal bread

Fresh dill (optional)

Preparation

Lightly toast the wholemeal bread. Spread fresh cheese on toast. Arrange the smoked salmon on top and garnish with a few sprigs of fresh dill. Tips, Try different types of fresh cheese and smoked salmon to vary the flavors Accompaniments: You can accompany your breakfasts with a cup of green tea or a coffee.

Estimated nutritional values (per serving):

Calories: 200-250 kcal

Protein: 25-30g

Carbohydrates: 15-20g

Fat: 10-15g

STABILIZATION PHASE

PROTEIN OMELETTE WITH VEGETABLES

Preparation time: 10 minutes

Cooking time: 15-20 minutes

Doses: 1 person

Ingredients:

2 eggs

50g of fresh spinach

30g of cherry tomatoes

15g of champignon mushrooms

1 clove of garlic

Salt, pepper and aromatic herbs

to taste (oregano, basil)

Preparation:

In a non-stick pan, lightly fry the garlic with a drizzle of oil. Add the sliced mushrooms and cook until golden brown. Add the spinach and the cherry tomatoes cut in half. Cook for a few minutes until the vegetables are wilted. Beat the eggs in a bowl, add salt, pepper and your favorite herbs. Pour the eggs over the vegetables in the pan and cook over medium heat, covering with a lid. When the egg is set, turn the omelette and cook the other side too.

Estimated nutritional values (per serving):

Calories: 200-250 kcal

Protein: 25-30g

Carbohydrates: 5-7g

Fat: 10-12g

GREEK YOGURT WITH NUTS AND SEEDS

Preparation time: 5 minutes

Cooking time: Not necessary

Doses: 1 person

Ingredients:

150g of Greek yogurt

30g of mixed nuts

(almonds, walnuts, hazelnuts)

1 tablespoon chia seeds

Fresh fruit of the season

(to taste, such as blueberries or strawberries)

Preparation:

Pour the Greek yogurt into a bowl. Add the coarsely chopped nuts, chia seeds and chopped fresh fruit. Mix delicately and sweeten with a teaspoon of honey if desired. Tips: Seasonal fruit: Choose seasonal fruit for a higher intake of vitamins and minerals.

Estimated nutritional values (per serving):

Calories: 250-300 kcal

Protein: 20-25g

Carbohydrates: 10-15g

Fat: 15-20g

RECIPES APPETIZERS

ATTACK PHASE

STUFFED EGGS WITH TUNA AND PARSLEY

Preparation time: 15 minutes

Cooking time: 10 minutes

Doses: 1 person

Ingredients:

1 egg

1 can of natural tuna (80 g)

1 tablespoon chopped parsley

1 tablespoon Greek yogurt

1/2 clove garlic, minced (optional)

Salt and Pepper To Taste

Preparation:

Cook the egg in boiling water for 10 minutes. Drain it and cool it under cold running water. Peel the egg and cut it in half lengthwise. Remove the yolk and place it in a bowl. Mash the egg yolk with a fork. Add the tuna, parsley, yogurt, garlic (if using), salt and pepper. Mix well until a homogeneous mixture is obtained. Fill the egg cavities with the tuna mixture. Serve immediately or store in the refrigerator for up to 2 days.

Nutritional values (per serving):

Calories: 150 kcal

Protein: 15 gr

Fat: 8 gr

Carbohydrates: 2 gr

BEEF CARPACCIO WITH ARUGULA AND PARMESAN FLAKES

Preparation time: 10 minutes

Cooking time: 0 minutes

Doses: 1 person

Ingredients:

100g of beef

lean (e.g. fillet, silverside)

50 g of Arugula

20 g of parmesan flakes

Extra virgin olive oil to taste

Lemon juice to taste

Salt and Pepper To Taste

Preparation:

Thinly slice the beef with a sharp knife or slicer. Arrange the slices of meat on a serving plate. Season with extra virgin olive oil, lemon juice, salt and pepper. Add the Arugula and parmesan flakes. Serve immediately.

Nutritional values (per serving):

Calories: 250 kcal

Protein: 25 gr

Fat: 15 gr

Carbohydrates: 1 g

GRILLED PRAWNS SKEWERS WITH LEMON

Preparation time: 10 minutes

Cooking time: 57 minutes

Doses: 1 person

Ingredients:

100g of cleaned fresh prawns

1/2 lemon

1/2 tablespoon of oil

extra virgin olive oil

Salt and Pepper To Taste

Preparation:

Wash the prawns and dry them with absorbent paper. Thread the prawns onto a wooden skewer. Drizzle the prawns with extra virgin olive oil, salt and pepper. Grill shrimp for 57 minutes per side, or until browned and cooked through. Serve the shrimp with lemon wedges.

Nutritional values (per serving):

Calories: 125 kcal

Protein: 15 gr

Fat: 5 gr

Carbohydrates: 0 gr

CHICKEN SALAD WITH CELERY AND MUSTARD

Preparation time: 15 minutes

Cooking time: 20 minutes

Doses: 1 person

Ingredients:

150 g of chicken breast

grilled or boiled

1 stalk of celery

1 tablespoon Greek yogurt

1 teaspoon of

Dijon mustard

Salt and Pepper To Taste

Preparation:

Cut the chicken breast into cubes. Wash the celery and cut it into thin slices. In a bowl, mix the chicken, celery, yogurt, mustard, salt and pepper. Serve the salad immediately. You can add other ingredients to the salad, such as tomatoes, cucumbers or olives. You can prepare the salad in advance and store it in the refrigerator for up to 2 days.

Nutritional values (per serving):

Calories: 300 kcal

Protein: 35 gr

Fat: 15 gr

Carbohydrates: 5 gr

SMOKED SALMON CANAPES WITH CUCUMBER

Preparation time: 5 minutes

Cooking time: 0 minutes

Doses: 1 person

Ingredients:

1 slice of wholemeal bread

50 g of smoked salmon

1/4 of a cucumber

Chopped parsley (optional)

Salt and Pepper To Taste

Preparation:

Toast wholemeal bread. Arrange the smoked salmon on the bread. Slice the cucumber thinly and arrange it on the salmon. Sprinkle with chopped parsley (optional). Salt and pepper to taste.

Nutritional values (per serving):

Calories: 250 kcal

Protein: 25 gr

Fat: 12 gr

Carbohydrates: 5 gr

GRILLED COURGETTES WITH FRESH TOMATO SAUCE

Preparation time: 15 minutes

Cooking time: 10 minutes

Doses: 1 person

Ingredients:

1 medium courgette

1 ripe tomato

1 tablespoon of oil

extra virgin olive oil

Chopped fresh basil

Salt and Pepper To Taste

Preparation:

Wash the courgette and cut it into slices about 1 cm thick. Grill the courgettes for 57 minutes per side, or until golden and tender. In the meantime, prepare the tomato sauce: cut the tomato into small pieces and place it in a bowl. Add the extra virgin olive oil, chopped basil, salt and pepper. Mix well. Serve the grilled courgettes with the fresh tomato sauce. You can add other ingredients to the tomato sauce, such as onion, garlic or chili pepper. If you prefer, you can cook the courgettes in the oven instead of on the grill.

Nutritional values (per serving):

Calories: 150 kcal

Protein: 10 gr

Fat: 8 gr

Carbohydrates: 5 gr

TOMATOES STUFFED WITH RICOTTA AND BASIL

Preparation time: 15 minutes

Cooking time: 15 minutes

Doses: 1 person

Ingredients:

10 cherry tomatoes

50 g of ricotta

1 tablespoon basil

fresh chopped

Salt and Pepper To Taste

Extra virgin olive oil

olive (optional)

Preparation:

Wash the cherry tomatoes and cut them in half lengthwise. Remove the seeds and pulp from the cherry tomatoes with a teaspoon. In a bowl, mix the ricotta, chopped basil, salt and pepper. Fill the cherry tomatoes with the ricotta mixture. Drizzle the cherry tomatoes with extra virgin olive oil (optional). Cook the cherry tomatoes in a preheated oven at 180°C for 15 minutes, or until they are golden.

Nutritional values (per serving):

Calories: 150 kcal

Protein: 15 gr

Fat: 8 gr

Carbohydrates: 5 gr

ROASTED PEPPERS STUFFED WITH TUNA AND CAPERS

Preparation time: 20 minutes

Cooking time: 30 minutes

Doses: 1 person

Ingredients:

1 red pepper

50 g of natural tuna

1 tablespoon capers

1 tablespoon of oil

extra virgin olive oil

Chopped parsley (optional)

Salt and Pepper To Taste

Preparation:

Wash the pepper and cut it in half lengthwise. Remove the seeds and the white part of the pepper. Cook the peppers in a preheated oven at 180°C for 30 minutes, or until they are soft. In the meantime, prepare the filling: in a bowl, crumble the tuna, add the capers, extra virgin olive oil, chopped parsley (optional), salt and pepper. Mix well. When the peppers are cooked, stuff them with the tuna mixture. Serve the peppers hot or cold. You can add other ingredients to the filling, such as olives, dried tomatoes or onion. Nutritional values (per serving):

Calories: 250 kcal

Protein: 25 gr

Fat: 15 gr

Carbohydrates: 5 gr

MOZZARELLA SKEWERS WITH TOMATOES

Preparation time: 10 minutes

Cooking time: 0 minutes

Doses: 1 person

Ingredients:

5 cherry tomatoes

5 morsels of mozzarella

Fresh basil (optional)

Extra virgin olive oil

olive (optional)

Salt and Pepper To Taste

Preparation:

Wash the cherry tomatoes and cut them in half. Drain the mozzarella and cut it into cubes. Thread the cherry tomatoes and mozzarella cubes alternately onto a wooden skewer. Decorate with fresh basil leaves (optional). Drizzle with extra virgin olive oil (optional). Salt and pepper to taste. You can use cherry tomatoes of different varieties and colors to make the skewers more colorful. If you prefer, you can use light or low-fat mozzarella.

Nutritional values (per serving):

Calories: 200 kcal

Protein: 20 gr

Fat: 12 gr

Carbohydrates: 5 gr

CRUISE PHASE

CHICKEN SALAD WITH GRILLED VEGETABLES

Preparation time: 20 minutes

Cooking time: 15 minutes

Doses: 1 person

Ingredients:

150g of chicken breast

grilled or boiled

1 medium courgette

1 medium aubergine

1 red pepper

1 tablespoon of oil

extra virgin olive oil

Chopped fresh basil

Salt and Pepper To Taste

Preparation:

Wash the vegetables and cut them into slices. Grill vegetables for 57 minutes per side, or until golden and tender. Cut the chicken breast into cubes. In a bowl, mix the chicken, grilled vegetables, extra virgin olive oil, chopped basil, salt and pepper. Serve the salad immediately.

Nutritional values (per serving):

Calories: 350 kcal

Protein: 40 gr

Fat: 15 gr

Carbohydrates: 10 gr

SMOKED SALMON MOUSSE WITH GREEK YOGURT

Preparation time: 10 minutes

Cooking time: 0 minutes

Doses: 1 person

Ingredients:

50 g of smoked salmon

100g of Greek yogurt

1 tablespoon lemon juice

Chives

chopped (optional)

Salt and Pepper To Taste

Preparation:

Blend the smoked salmon, Greek yogurt, lemon juice, salt and pepper in a blender until smooth. Decorate with chopped chives (optional). Serve the mousse immediately. You can use other types of smoked fish, such as trout or mackerel. If you prefer, you can use low-fat or light Greek yogurt. You can add other ingredients to the mousse, such as avocado, cream cheese or spices

Nutritional values (per serving):

Calories: 250 kcal

Protein: 30 gr

Fat: 12 gr

Carbohydrates: 5 gr

BEET CARPACCIO WITH RICOTTA

Preparation time: 15 minutes

Cooking time: 0 minutes

Doses: 1 person

Ingredients:

100 g of pre-cooked beetroot

50 g of ricotta

1 walnut

Chopped parsley

(optional)

Salt and Pepper To Taste

Extra virgin olive oil

olive (optional)

Preparation:

Peel the pre-cooked beetroot and cut it into thin slices with a mandolin or sharp knife. Arrange the beetroot slices on a serving plate. Crumble the ricotta over the beetroot slices. Chop the walnut and sprinkle it on the ricotta. Sprinkle with chopped parsley (optional). Salt and pepper to taste. Drizzle with extra virgin olive oil (optional).

Nutritional values (per serving):

Calories: 250 kcal

Protein: 20 gr

Fat: 15 gr

Carbohydrates: 10 gr

SHRIMP AND COURGETTE SKEWERS

Preparation time: 20 minutes

Cooking time: 10 minutes

Doses: 1 person

Ingredients:

100g of cleaned fresh prawns

1 medium courgette

1 tablespoon of oil

extra virgin olive oil

Chopped fresh basil

Salt and Pepper To Taste

Preparation:

Wash the prawns and dry them with absorbent paper. Wash the courgette and cut it into rounds. Thread the prawns and courgette slices alternately onto a wooden skewer. Drizzle the skewers with extra virgin olive oil, salt and pepper. Grill the skewers for 57 minutes per side, or until the shrimp are golden brown and cooked through. Decorate with chopped fresh basil. You can use other types of vegetables for the skewers, such as peppers, eggplant or onions. If you prefer, you can cook the skewers in the oven instead of on the grill.

Nutritional values (per serving):

Calories: 300 kcal

Protein: 35 gr

Fat: 15 gr

Carbohydrates: 5 gr

STUFFED EGGS WITH TUNA AND GREEK YOGURT

Preparation time: 15 minutes

Cooking time: 10 minutes

Doses: 1 person

Ingredients:

2 eggs

50 g of natural tuna

2 tablespoons Greek yogurt

1 tablespoon capers

Parsley

chopped (optional)

Salt and Pepper To Taste

Preparation:

Cook the eggs in boiling water for 10 minutes. Drain them and cool them under cold water. Peel the eggs and cut them in half lengthwise. Remove the egg yolks and place them in a bowl. Chop the tuna and add it to the egg yolks. Add the Greek yogurt, capers, chopped parsley (optional), salt and pepper. Mix well. Fill the egg cavities with the tuna mixture. Serve immediately.

Nutritional values (per serving):

Calories: 250 kcal

Protein: 25 gr

Fat: 15 gr

Carbohydrates: 5 gr

SEAFOOD SALAD WITH VEGETABLES

Preparation time: 20 minutes

Cooking time: 10 minutes

Doses: 1 person

Ingredients:

100g of cleaned fresh prawns

100g of calamari

1 medium courgette

1 tomato

1 tablespoon of oil

extra virgin olive oil

Chopped fresh basil

Salt and Pepper To Taste

Preparation:

Wash the prawns and squid and dry them with absorbent paper. Cook the prawns and calamari in boiling water for 5 minutes. Drain them and cool them. Wash the courgette and cut it into thin slices. Cut the tomato into small pieces. In a bowl, mix the prawns, calamari, courgette, tomato, extra virgin olive oil, chopped basil, salt and pepper. Serve the salad immediately. You can use other types of fish and seafood for the salad. If you prefer, you can cook the shrimp and calamari on the grill or steam instead of boiling water.

Nutritional values (per serving):

Calories: 350 kcal

Protein: 40 gr

Fat: 15 gr

Carbohydrates: 10 gr

SALMON CARPACCIO WITH YOGURT AND CHIVE SAUCE

Preparation time: 15 minutes

Cooking time: 0 minutes

Doses: 1 person

Ingredients:

100g of smoked salmon

100g of Greek yogurt

1 tablespoon lemon juice

1 tablespoon chopped chives

Salt and Pepper To Taste

Preparation:

Arrange the smoked salmon slices on a serving plate. In a bowl, mix the Greek yogurt, lemon juice, chopped chives, salt and pepper. Pour the yogurt sauce over the smoked salmon. Serve immediately.

Nutritional values (per serving):

Calories: 300 kcal

Protein: 35 gr

Fat: 15 gr

Carbohydrates: 5 gr

COURGETTE FRITTERS WITH MINT AND LEMON

Preparation time: 20 minutes

Cooking time: 10 minutes

Doses: 1 person

Ingredients:

1 medium courgette

1 egg

2 tablespoons oat flour

1 tablespoon chopped fresh mint

1 tablespoon lemon juice

Salt and Pepper To Taste

Extra virgin olive oil

olive for frying

Preparation:

Wash the courgette and grate it. In a bowl, mix the grated courgette, egg, oat flour, chopped mint, lemon juice, salt and pepper. Heat the extra virgin olive oil in a non-stick pan. Pour a spoonful of pancake mixture into the pan and cook for 23 minutes per side, or until golden brown. Drain the pancakes on absorbent paper. Serve immediately.

Nutritional values (per serving):

Calories: 250 kcal

Protein: 15 gr

Fat: 15 gr

Carbohydrates: 15 gr

PEPPER ROLLS WITH TUNA AND BLACK OLIVES

Preparation time: 25 minutes

Cooking time: 15 minutes

Doses: 1 person

Ingredients:

1 red pepper

50 g of natural tuna

10 black olives

1 tablespoon capers

1 tablespoon of

chopped parsley

Salt and Pepper To Taste

Extra virgin olive oil

olive (optional)

Preparation:

Wash the pepper and cut it into strips about 2 cm wide. Cook the pepper strips in boiling water for 5 minutes. Drain them and cool them. Chop the tuna and mix it with the black olives, capers, chopped parsley, salt and pepper. Place a spoonful of tuna mixture on each pepper strip. Roll the pepper strips to form rolls. Drizzle the rolls with extra virgin olive oil (optional). Serve immediately. You can add other ingredients to the tuna mixture, such as cream cheese or spices.

Nutritional values (per serving):

Calories: 350 kcal

Protein: 35 gr

Fat: 20 gr

Carbohydrates: 5 gr

CONSOLIDATION PHASE

QUINOA SALAD WITH GRILLED VEGETABLES AND FETA

Preparation time: 30 minutes

Cooking time: 20 minutes

Doses: 1 person

Ingredients:

50g of quinoa

1 medium courgette

1 medium aubergine

1 red pepper

50 g of feta

1 tablespoon of oil

extra virgin olive oil

Chopped fresh basil

Salt and Pepper To Taste

Preparation:

Rinse the quinoa under running water. Cook the quinoa in boiling salted water for 15 minutes. Drain it and cool it. Wash the vegetables and cut them into slices. Grill vegetables for 57 minutes per side, or until golden and tender. Cut the feta into cubes. In a bowl, mix the quinoa, grilled vegetables, feta, extra virgin olive oil, chopped basil, salt and pepper. Serve the salad immediately.

Nutritional values (per serving):

Calories: 450 kcal

Protein: 30 gr

Fat: 20 gr

Carbohydrates: 35 gr

WHOLE WHOLE BRUSCHETTA WITH TOMATOES AND FRESH BASIL

Preparation time: 15 minutes

Cooking time: 10 minutes

Doses: 4 bruschettas

Ingredients:

4 slices of wholemeal bread

200g of cherry tomatoes

10 fresh basil leaves

1 clove of garlic

2 tablespoons of oil

extra virgin olive oil

Salt and Pepper To Taste

Preparation:

Cut the cherry tomatoes into small pieces. Chop the fresh basil. Fry the chopped garlic in extra virgin olive oil for 1 minute. Add the cherry tomatoes and cook for 5 minutes. Salt and pepper to taste. Toast the slices of wholemeal bread. Spread the bread slices with the cherry tomato mixture. Decorate with fresh basil leaves. Serve the bruschetta immediately. You can use other types of vegetables for the bruschetta, such as peppers, aubergines or onions.

Nutritional values (per serving):

Calories: 250 kcal

Protein: 10 gr

Fat: 15 gr

Carbohydrates: 25 gr

CAPRESE WITH TOMATO, LIGHT MOZZARELLA AND BASIL

Preparation time: 10 minutes

Cooking time: 0 minutes

Doses: 1 person

Ingredients:

1 ripe tomato

100g of light mozzarella

5 fresh basil leaves

Extra virgin olive oil

olive (optional)

Salt and Pepper To Taste

Preparation:

Wash the tomato and cut it into slices. Cut the light mozzarella into slices. Arrange the tomato and mozzarella slices on a plate alternating them. Decorate with fresh basil leaves. Drizzle with extra virgin olive oil (optional). Salt and pepper to taste. Serve the caprese immediately.

Nutritional values (per serving):

Calories: 250 kcal

Protein: 25 gr

Fat: 15 gr

Carbohydrates: 5 gr

WHOLE BREAD CANAPÉS WITH AVOCADO AND SALMON SMOKED

Preparation time: 15 minutes

Cooking time: 0 minutes

Servings: 2 canapés

Ingredients:

2 slices of wholemeal bread

1/2 ripe avocado

50 g of smoked salmon

Lemon juice (optional)

Salt and Pepper To Taste

Preparation:

Toast the slices of wholemeal bread. Mash the avocado with a fork and spread it on the toast. Arrange the smoked salmon on the bread with the avocado. Drizzle with lemon juice (optional). Salt and pepper to taste. Serve the canapés immediately. You can use other types of bread for canapés, such as rye bread or cereal bread. If you prefer, you can bake the avocado for 10 minutes before mashing it.

Nutritional values (per serving):

Calories: 350 kcal

Protein: 30 gr

Fat: 20 gr

Carbohydrates: 20 gr

BUCKWHEAT FRITTERS WITH COURGETTES AND PARMESAN

Preparation time: 20 minutes

Cooking time: 10 minutes

Servings: 4 pancakes

Ingredients:

50 g of buckwheat flour

1 medium courgette

30 g of grated parmesan

1 egg

1 tablespoon of skimmed milk

1 tablespoon of oil

extra virgin olive oil

Salt and Pepper To Taste

Preparation:

Wash the courgette and grate it. In a bowl, mix the buckwheat flour, grated parmesan, egg, skimmed milk, extra virgin olive oil, salt and pepper. Add the grated courgette and mix well. Heat the extra virgin olive oil in a non-stick pan. Pour a spoonful of pancake mixture into the pan and cook for 23 minutes per side, or until golden brown. Drain the pancakes on absorbent paper. Serve the pancakes immediately.

Nutritional values (per serving):

Calories: 250 kcal

Protein: 15 gr

Fat: 15 gr

Carbohydrates: 20 gr

LENTIL SALAD WITH ROASTED PEPPERS AND TUNA

Preparation time: 30 minutes

Cooking time: 20 minutes

Doses: 1 person

Ingredients:

50 g of dried lentils

1 red pepper

50 g of natural tuna

1 tablespoon of oil

extra virgin olive oil

Red onion (optional)

Chopped parsley (optional)

Salt and Pepper To Taste

Preparation:

Rinse the lentils under running water. Cook the lentils in boiling salted water for 20 minutes. Drain them and cool them. Wash the pepper and cut it into strips. Bake or grill the pepper strips for 10 minutes, or until soft. Chop the tuna. In a bowl, mix the lentils, roasted peppers, tuna, extra virgin olive oil, salt and pepper. Add chopped red onion and chopped parsley (optional). Serve the salad immediately. You can use other types of legumes for the salad, such as chickpeas or beans.

Nutritional values (per serving):

Calories: 400 kcal

Protein: 35 gr

Fat: 20 gr

Carbohydrates: 25 gr

GRILLED AUBERGINE ROLLS WITH COOKED HAM AND LIGHT CHEESE

Preparation time: 25 minutes

Cooking time: 15 minutes

Doses: 2 rolls

Ingredients:

1 medium aubergine

50 g of cooked ham

50 g of light cheese

Fresh basil (optional)

Extra virgin olive oil

olive (optional)

Salt and Pepper To Taste

Preparation:

Wash the aubergine and cut it into thin longitudinal slices. Grill the aubergine slices for 5 minutes per side, or until soft. Drain them and cool them. Arrange a slice of cooked ham on each slice of grilled aubergine. Add a slice of light cheese. Roll up the aubergine slices to form rolls. Decorate with fresh basil (optional). Drizzle with extra virgin olive oil (optional). Salt and pepper to taste. Serve the rolls immediately.

Nutritional values (per serving):

Calories: 300 kcal

Protein: 25 gr

Fat: 15 gr

Carbohydrates: 10 gr

WHOLE BREAD CROUTTONS WITH RICOTTA CREAM AND DRIED TOMATOES

Preparation time: 15 minutes

Cooking time: 0 minutes

Servings: 4 croutons

Ingredients:

4 slices of wholemeal bread

100 g of ricotta

5 dried tomatoes

Fresh basil (optional)

Extra virgin olive oil

olive (optional)

Salt and Pepper To Taste

Preparation:

Toast the slices of wholemeal bread. In a bowl, mix the ricotta, chopped dried tomatoes, chopped fresh basil (optional), extra virgin olive oil (optional), salt and pepper. Spread the ricotta cream on the wholemeal bread croutons. Serve the croutons immediately.

Nutritional values (per serving):

Calories: 250 kcal

Protein: 15 gr

Fat: 15 gr

Carbohydrates: 20 gr

CHICKEN SALAD WITH MANGO, AVOCADO AND SUNFLOWER SEEDS

Preparation time: 20 minutes

Cooking time: 10 minutes (for chicken)

Doses: 1 person

Ingredients:

100g of chicken breast

1/2 ripe mango

1/2 ripe avocado

1 tablespoon sunflower seeds

Lime juice (optional)

Extra virgin olive oil

olive (optional)

Salt and Pepper To Taste

Preparation:

Cook the chicken breast on the grill or in a pan for 10 minutes. Cut the chicken into small pieces. Cut the mango into small pieces. Cut the avocado into small pieces. In a bowl, mix the chicken, mango, avocado, sunflower seeds, lime juice (optional), extra virgin olive oil (optional), salt and pepper. Serve the salad immediately. You can use other fruits for the salad, such as pineapple or papaya. If you prefer, you can cook the chicken in the oven. Nutritional values (per portion):

Calories: 450 kcal

Protein: 35 gr

Fat: 25 gr

Carbohydrates: 15 gr

STABILIZATION PHASE

GREEK SALAD WITH TOMATOES, CUCUMBERS, PEPPERS, OLIVES AND FETA

Preparation time: 20 minutes

Cooking time: 0 minutes

Doses: 1 person

Ingredients:

1 ripe tomato

1/2 cucumber

1/2 green or red pepper

10 black olives

50 g of feta

1 tablespoon extra virgin olive oil

Fresh oregano (optional)

Salt and Pepper To Taste

Preparation:

Wash the tomato, cucumber and pepper. Cut the tomato into slices, the cucumber into pieces and the pepper into strips. Arrange the vegetables on a serving plate. Add the black olives and crumbled feta. Drizzle with extra virgin olive oil. Sprinkle with fresh oregano (optional). Salt and pepper to taste. Serve the salad immediately.

Nutritional values (per serving):

Calories: 350 kcal

Protein: 25 gr

Fat: 20 gr

Carbohydrates: 10 gr

AVOCADO CARPACCIO WITH PRAWNS AND MANGO

Preparation time: 20 minutes

Cooking time: 0 minutes

Doses: 1 person

Ingredients:

1/2 ripe avocado

5 cleaned prawns

1/2 ripe mango

1 tablespoon lime juice

1 tablespoon of oil

extra virgin olive oil

Sesame seeds (optional)

Salt and Pepper To Taste

Preparation:

Cut the avocado into thin slices. Arrange the avocado slices on a serving plate. Chop the prawns and arrange them on the avocado. Cut the mango into thin slices and arrange them on the prawns. Drizzle with lime juice and extra virgin olive oil. Sprinkle with sesame seeds (optional). Salt and pepper to taste. Serve the carpaccio immediately.

Nutritional values (per serving):

Calories: 400 kcal

Protein: 30 gr

Fat: 25 gr

Carbohydrates: 15 gr

WHOLE WHOLE BRUSCHETTE WITH CHERRY TOMATOES, BASIL AND BUFFALO MOZZARELLA

Preparation time: 15 minutes

Cooking time: 10 minutes

(to toast bread)

Doses: 4 bruschettas

Ingredients:

4 slices of wholemeal bread

200g of cherry tomatoes

10 fresh basil leaves

100g of buffalo mozzarella

Extra virgin olive oil

olive (optional)

Salt and Pepper To Taste

Preparation:

Toast the slices of wholemeal bread. Wash the cherry tomatoes and cut them into small pieces. Chop the fresh basil. Cut the buffalo mozzarella into slices. Arrange the cherry tomatoes, chopped basil and buffalo mozzarella on the toasted bread slices. Drizzle with extra virgin olive oil (optional). Salt and pepper to taste. Serve the bruschetta immediately.

Nutritional values (per serving):

Calories: 350 kcal

Protein: 25 gr

Fat: 20 gr

Carbohydrates: 15 gr

WHOLE BREAD CANAPÉS WITH CHICKPEA HUMMUS AND GRILLED VEGETABLES

Preparation time: 25 minutes

Cooking time: 15 minutes

(for grilling vegetables)

Servings: 2 canapés

Ingredients:

2 slices of wholemeal bread

100g of boiled chickpeas

1/2 aubergine

1/2 red pepper

1 tablespoon lemon juice

1 clove of garlic

1 tablespoon tahini

Salt and Pepper To Taste

Preparation:

Toast the slices of wholemeal bread. Wash the aubergine and pepper. Cut the aubergine into slices and the pepper into strips. Grill the vegetables for 10 minutes, or until soft. In a food processor, blend the boiled chickpeas, grilled vegetables, lemon juice, garlic, tahini, extra virgin olive oil (optional), salt and pepper until creamy. Spread the chickpea hummus on the toasted bread slices. Serve the canapés immediately.

Nutritional values (per serving):

Calories: 400 kcal

Protein: 30 gr

Fat: 25 gr

Carbohydrates: 15 gr

ROLLS OF RAW HAM WITH MELON AND FRESH CHEESE

Preparation time: 15 minutes

Cooking time: 0 minutes

Doses: 4 rolls

Ingredients:

4 slices of raw ham

1/4 of a ripe melon

100g of fresh cheese

(like ricotta or robiola)

Fresh basil (optional)

Salt and Pepper To Taste

Preparation:

Cut the melon into thin slices. Spread the fresh cheese on the melon slices. Arrange a slice of raw ham on each slice of melon with fresh cheese. Roll up the melon slices to form rolls. Decorate with fresh basil (optional). Salt and pepper to taste. Serve the rolls immediately.

Nutritional values (per serving):

Calories: 300 kcal

Protein: 20 gr

Fat: 15 gr

Carbohydrates: 15 gr

QUINOA FRITTERS WITH SPINACH AND LIGHT CHEESE

Preparation time: 20 minutes

Cooking time: 10 minutes

Servings: 4 pancakes

Ingredients:

50g of quinoa

100g of spinach

50 g of cheese

light grated

1 egg

1 tablespoon of skimmed milk

1 tablespoon of oil

extra virgin olive oil

Salt and Pepper To Taste

Preparation:

Rinse the quinoa under running water. Cook the quinoa in boiling salted water for 15 minutes. Drain it and cool it. Wash the spinach and boil them in a little boiling water for 2 minutes. Remove the spinach and squeeze it well. In a bowl, mix the quinoa, chopped spinach, grated light cheese, egg, skimmed milk, extra virgin olive oil, salt and pepper. Heat the extra virgin olive oil in a non-stick pan. Pour a spoonful of pancake mixture into the pan and cook for 23 minutes per side, or until golden brown. Drain the pancakes on absorbent paper. Serve the pancakes immediately. Nutritional values (per serving): Calories: 250 kcal

Protein: 20 gr

Fat: 10 gr

Carbohydrates: 20 gr

TUNA SALAD WITH CANNELLINI BEANS, RED ONION AND PARSLEY

Preparation time: 20 minutes

Cooking time: 0 minutes

Doses: 1 person

Ingredients:

120g of natural tuna

100g of boiled cannellini beans

1/2 red onion

Fresh parsley

Extra virgin olive oil

olive (optional)

Lemon juice (optional)

Salt and Pepper To Taste

Preparation:

Chop the tuna. Rinse the cannellini beans under running water. Cut the red onion into thin slices. Chop the fresh parsley. In a bowl, mix the tuna, cannellini beans, red onion, fresh parsley, extra virgin olive oil (optional), lemon juice (optional), salt and pepper. Serve the salad immediately.

Nutritional values (per serving):

Calories: 400 kcal

Protein: 35 gr

Fat: 20 gr

Carbohydrates: 25 gr

WHOLE BREAD CROUTTONS WITH CREAM CHEESE AND COOKED HAM

Preparation time: 15 minutes

Cooking time: 0 minutes

Servings: 4 croutons

Ingredients:

4 slices of wholemeal bread

100g of fresh cheese

(like ricotta or robiola)

50 g of cooked ham

Fresh basil (optional)

Extra virgin olive oil

olive (optional)

Salt and Pepper To Taste

Preparation:

Toast the slices of wholemeal bread. In a bowl, mix the fresh cheese, chopped cooked ham, chopped fresh basil (optional), extra virgin olive oil (optional), salt and pepper. Spread the cream cheese and ham on the wholemeal bread croutons. Serve the croutons immediately.

Nutritional values (per serving):

Calories: 250 kcal

Protein: 20 gr

Fat: 15 gr

Carbohydrates: 15 gr

CHICKEN SALAD WITH AVOCADO, CORN AND GREEK YOGURT SAUCE

Preparation time: 25 minutes

Cooking time: 10 minutes

Doses: 1 person

Ingredients:

100g of chicken breast

1/2 ripe avocado

1 tablespoon of corn

100g of Greek yogurt

Lime juice (optional)

Extra virgin olive oil

olive (optional)

Salt and Pepper To Taste

Preparation:

Cook the chicken breast on the grill or in a pan for 10 minutes. Cut the chicken into small pieces. Cut the avocado into small pieces. In a bowl, mix the chicken, avocado, corn, Greek yogurt, lime juice (optional), extra virgin olive oil (optional), salt, and pepper. Serve the salad immediately. You can add other ingredients to the salad, such as olives, tomatoes or herbs.

Nutritional values (per serving):

Calories: 450 kcal

Protein: 40 gr

Fat: 25 gr

Carbohydrates: 10 gr

RECIPES
FIRST DISHES

ATTACK PHASE

KONJAC PENNE WITH GENOVESE PESTO

Preparation time: 10 minutes

Cooking time: 5 minutes

Doses: 1 person

Ingredients:

100g of konjac pens

50 g of Genoese pesto

25 g of cherry tomatoes

Fresh basil (optional)

Salt and Pepper To Taste

Preparation:

Rinse the konjac pens: Rinse the konjac pens under running water to remove any preservative liquid. Cook the konjac penne: Cook the konjac penne in boiling water for 23 minutes. Drain the konjac penne: Drain the konjac penne and drain well. Season the konjac penne: In a bowl, season the konjac penne with the Genoese pesto. Add the cherry tomatoes: Cut the cherry tomatoes in half and add them to the seasoned konjac penne.

Decorate with fresh basil (optional): If desired, decorate the dish with fresh basil leaves. Salt and pepper to taste: Salt and pepper to taste. Serve the konjac penne with Genoese pesto immediately, piping hot.

Nutritional values (per serving):

Calories: 125 kcal

Protein: 10 gr

Fat: 7.5 gr

Carbohydrates: 2.5 gr

CAULIFLOWER RISOTTO WITH PORCINI MUSHROOMS

Preparation time: 20 minutes

Cooking time: 15 minutes

Doses: 1 person

Ingredients:

1/4 of cauliflower

50 g of porcini mushrooms

1/2 onion

25 g of grated parmesan

Vegetable broth (optional)

Extra virgin olive oil

Salt and Pepper To Taste

Preparation:

Cut the cauliflower: Cut the cauliflower into florets. Wash the porcini mushrooms: Wash the porcini mushrooms and cut them into slices. Chop the onion: Finely chop the onion. Fry the onion: In a pan, heat the extra virgin olive oil and fry the onion until it becomes transparent. Add the porcini mushrooms: Add the chopped porcini mushrooms to the onion and cook them for 23 minutes. Add the cauliflower: Add the cauliflower florets to the pan and cook them for about 5 minutes. Add vegetable broth (optional): If necessary, add a little vegetable broth to help cook the cauliflower.

Cook the cauliflower: Cook the cauliflower until soft, about 10 minutes. Stir in the grated parmesan: Remove the pan from the heat and stir in the risotto with the grated parmesan. Salt and pepper to taste: Salt and pepper to taste. Serve immediately: Serve the cauliflower risotto with porcini mushrooms immediately, piping hot.

Nutritional values (per serving):

Calories: 150 kcal

Protein: 12.5 gr

Fat: 7.5 gr

Carbohydrates: 5 gr

ZUCCHINI LASAGNA WITH TURKEY SAUCE

Preparation time: 40 minutes

Cooking time: 45 minutes

Doses: 1 person

Ingredients

200 g of courgettes

200g of minced turkey

400 g of peeled tomatoes

1 onion

1 clove of garlic

Fresh basil

30 g of parmesan

light grated (optional)

2 tablespoons extra virgin olive oil

Salt and Pepper To Taste

Preparation:

Prepare the ragù (20 minutes): Chop onion and garlic. Saute the onion in olive oil until transparent. Add garlic and cook for 1 minute. Add ground turkey and cook crumbling it for 10 minutes. Add peeled tomatoes, basil, salt and pepper. Cook over low heat for 20 minutes, stirring. Prepare the courgettes (5 minutes): Wash and cut the courgettes into thin slices (3 mm). Assemble the lasagna (10 minutes): Spread a first layer of ragù in a non-stick pan. Cover with the courgette slices. Repeat layers, ending with ragù. Cover the pan with foil.

Bake in a preheated oven at 180°C for 30 minutes. Uncover the pan and sprinkle with parmesan (optional). Bake for a further 15 minutes until golden brown. Serve (10 minutes): Let the lasagna rest for 10 minutes before serving.

Nutritional values (per serving):

Calories: 450 kcal

Protein: 40 gr

Fat: 25 gr

Carbohydrates: 10 gr

CAULIFLOWER OMELETTE WITH TOMATO AND MOZZARELLA

Preparation time: 20 minutes

Cooking time: 20 minutes

Doses: 1 person

Ingredients:

200g of cauliflower

3 eggs

50 g of light mozzarella

100g of cherry tomatoes

Fresh basil

1 tablespoon of oil

extra virgin olive oil

Salt and Pepper To Taste

Preparation:

Prepare the cauliflower (10 minutes): Wash and cut the cauliflower into florets. Steam for 10 minutes until soft. Prepare the omelette (10 minutes): Beat the eggs with salt and pepper in a bowl. Heat the oil in a non-stick pan. Pour the egg mixture into the pan. Distribute evenly. Assemble the omelette (5 minutes): Arrange the cooked cauliflower, halved cherry tomatoes and sliced or grated mozzarella on the omelette. Cooking (15 minutes): Cover the pan with a lid. Cook over low heat for 15 minutes. Check for doneness and cook until golden brown. Serve (5 minutes): Enjoy the omelette hot. Nutritional values (per serving): Calories: 300 kcal

Protein: 25 gr

Fat: 15 gr

Carbohydrates: 10 gr

SCRAMBLED EGGS WITH SALMON AND SPINACH

Preparation time: 10 minutes

Cooking time: 5 minutes

Doses: 1 person

Ingredients:

2 eggs

100g of smoked salmon

100g of fresh spinach

1 tablespoon of oil

extra virgin olive oil

Salt and Pepper To Taste

Preparation:

Fry the oil: Heat the extra virgin olive oil in a non-stick pan.

Cook the spinach: Add the washed spinach and cook for a couple of minutes until wilted. Add the salmon: Add the smoked salmon cut into strips and cook for another minute. Beat the eggs: Beat the eggs in a bowl with a pinch of salt and pepper. Pour in the eggs: Pour the beaten eggs into the pan with the spinach and salmon. Cook the eggs: Cook the scrambled eggs over medium-low heat, stirring occasionally, until the desired consistency is reached. Serve: Serve the scrambled eggs with salmon and spinach immediately. Nutritional values (per serving):

Calories: 250 kcal

Protein: 25 gr

Fat: 15 gr

Carbohydrates: 0 gr

TUNA SALAD WITH TOMATOES AND OLIVES

Preparation time: 10 minutes

Cooking time: 0 minutes

Doses: 1 person

Ingredients:

120g of canned tuna

1 medium tomato

50 g of pitted black olives

1 tablespoon of oil

extra virgin olive oil

Fresh oregano (optional)

Salt and Pepper To Taste

Preparation:

Cut the tomato: Cut the tomato into small pieces. Chop the olives: Chop the black olives. Assemble the salad: In a bowl, combine the drained tuna, tomato, olives, extra virgin olive oil, fresh oregano (optional), salt and pepper. Mix the ingredients: Mix the ingredients well. Serve: Serve the tuna salad with tomatoes and olives chilled.

Nutritional values (per serving):

Calories: 200 kcal

Protein: 20 gr

Fat: 10 gr

Carbohydrates: 5 gr

OMELETTE WITH MUSHROOMS AND CHEESE

Preparation time: 10 minutes

Cooking time: 5 minutes

Doses: 1 person

Ingredients:

2 eggs

50 g of mushrooms

fresh (of your choice)

20 g of cheese

grated light

1 tablespoon butter

Salt and Pepper To Taste

Preparation:

Fry the butter: Fry the butter in a non-stick pan. Cook the mushrooms: Wash and slice the mushrooms. Add them to the pan and cook for about 5 minutes, or until tender. Beat the eggs: Beat the eggs in a bowl with a pinch of salt and pepper. Pour in the eggs: Pour the beaten eggs into the pan with the mushrooms. Sprinkle with cheese: Sprinkle with light grated cheese. Cook the omelette: Cook the omelette over medium-low heat, folding it in half when the edges begin to firm up. Serve the omelette with mushrooms and cheese piping hot.

Nutritional values (per serving):

Calories: 280 kcal

Protein: 22 gr

Fat: 20 gr

Carbohydrates: 2 gr

GRILLED CHICKEN SALAD WITH AVOCADO AND CUCUMBERS

Preparation time: 15 minutes

Cooking time: 10 minutes

Doses: 1 person

Ingredients:

150g of chicken breast

1/2 ripe avocado

1 medium cucumber

1 tablespoon of oil

extra virgin olive oil

Lemon juice (optional)

Salt and Pepper To Taste

Preparation:

Cook the chicken breast on the grill or in a non-stick pan for about 10 minutes per side, or until golden brown and cooked through. Cut the cucumber: Wash the cucumber and cut it into thin slices. Chop the avocado: Chop the ripe avocado into a bowl. Season the avocado: Drizzle the avocado with a drizzle of lemon juice (optional) to prevent it from blackening. Assemble the salad: In a large bowl, combine the sliced grilled chicken, the sliced cucumber, the chopped avocado, the extra virgin olive oil, salt and pepper to taste. Mix the ingredients: Mix the ingredients well to combine everything. Serve the grilled chicken salad with avocado and cucumbers chilled. Nutritional values (per serving):

Calories: 300 kcal, Protein: 30 gr

Fat: 18 g, Carbohydrates: 5 g

CRUISE PHASE

BRESAOLA SALAD WITH ARUGULA, PARMESAN AND MELON

Preparation time: 10 minutes

Cooking time: 0 minutes

Doses: 1 person

Ingredients:

100g of bresaola

100g of arugula

50 g of parmesan

150 g of melon

Extra virgin olive oil

Balsamic vinegar

Salt and Pepper To Taste

Preparation:

Cut the melon into slices and then into cubes. In a serving dish, arrange the arugula, sliced bresaola, diced melon and flaked parmesan. Drizzle the salad with a drizzle of extra virgin olive oil and balsamic vinegar. Add salt and pepper to taste. Serve the bresaola salad with rocket, parmesan and melon fresh.

Nutritional values (per serving):

Calories: 350 kcal

Protein: 30 gr

Fat: 15 gr

Carbohydrates: 5 gr

KONJAC SPAGHETTI WITH CLAMS AND TOMATOES

Preparation time: 15 minutes

Cooking time: 10 minutes

Doses: 1 person

Ingredients:

200g of konjac spaghetti

200g of clams

200g of cherry tomatoes

1 clove of garlic

1/2 glass of dry white wine

Fresh parsley

Extra virgin olive oil

Salt and Pepper To Taste

Preparation:

Rinse the clams carefully under running water to remove any impurities. In a pan, heat the extra virgin olive oil and fry the chopped garlic for a minute. Add the clams to the pan and deglaze with the white wine. Cover the pan and cook the clams for about 5 minutes, or until they open. Cut the cherry tomatoes in half and add them to the clams. Cook for another couple of minutes. Rinse and drain the konjac spaghetti. Add the drained konjac to the pan with the clams and cherry tomatoes. Mix well to combine everything. Add chopped fresh parsley, salt and pepper to taste. Serve the konjac spaghetti with clams and cherry tomatoes piping hot. Nutritional values (per serving):

Calories: 250 kcal, Protein: 25 gr

Fat: 10 g, Carbohydrates: 5 g

FENNEL CREAM
WITH SHRIMPS

Preparation time: 20 minutes

Cooking time: 30 minutes

Doses: 1 person

Ingredients:

200 g of fennel

1/2 onion

1/2 medium potato

350 ml of vegetable broth

100g of cleaned shrimps

Extra virgin olive oil

Salt and Pepper To Taste

Preparation:

Wash and clean the fennel, onion and potato. Cut the fennel into small pieces, the onion into slices and the potato into cubes. In a pan, heat the extra virgin olive oil and fry the onion for a couple of minutes. Add the fennel and potato and cook for about 5 minutes, stirring occasionally. Pour in the vegetable broth and bring to the boil. Cook for about 20 minutes, or until the fennel and potato are tender. Blend the mixture with a blender until you obtain a smooth cream. Add the shrimp to the cream and cook for another minute. Season with salt and pepper to taste. Serve the fennel cream with prawns piping hot. Nutritional values (per portion): Calories: 175 kcal, Protein: 15 gr

Fat: 7.5 gr

Carbohydrates: 5 gr

**LIGHT FISH SOUP WITH
MIXED VEGETABLES**

Preparation time: 30 minutes

Cooking time: 40 minutes

Doses: 1 person

Ingredients:

250 g of mixed fish (including

cod, sea bream, mackerel)

100 g of mixed vegetables (between

including carrots, courgettes, potatoes)

1/2 onion

1/4 clove of garlic

750 ml of vegetable broth

Extra virgin olive oil

Fresh parsley

Salt and Pepper To Taste

Preparation:

Wash and clean the fish. Cut the vegetables into small pieces. In a pan, heat the extra virgin olive oil and fry the chopped onion and garlic for a couple of minutes. Add the mixed vegetables and cook for about 5 minutes, stirring occasionally. Pour in the vegetable broth and bring to the boil. Cook for about 20 minutes, or until the vegetables are tender. Add the fish and cook for another 10 minutes, or until the fish is cooked through. Season with salt and pepper to taste. Sprinkle with chopped fresh parsley. Serve the light fish soup with mixed vegetables piping hot. Nutritional values (per serving):

Calories: 125 kcal

Protein: 15 gr

Fat: 5 gr

Carbohydrates: 2.5 g

TUNA AND MUSHROOM OMELETTE

Preparation time: 10 minutes

Cooking time: 15 minutes

Doses: 1 person

Ingredients:

2 eggs

70 g of natural tuna

50 g of fresh mixed mushrooms

1/2 small onion

1 tablespoon of oil

extra virgin olive oil

Salt and Pepper To Taste

Fresh parsley

chopped (optional)

Preparation:

Finely chop the onion. Wash and slice the mushrooms. Heat the oil in a non-stick pan. Fry the onion for a few minutes, until it softens. Add the mushrooms and cook for 57 minutes, stirring often. Add the drained and crumbled tuna. In a bowl, beat the eggs with a pinch of salt and pepper. Pour the egg mixture into the pan with the tuna and mushrooms. Cook the omelette over low heat for about 5 minutes, until the bottom has thickened. Fold the omelette in half and cook for another 23 minutes. and serve hot.

Nutritional values:

Calories: approximately 300 kcal

Protein: approximately 35 g

Fat: approximately 15 g

Carbohydrates: approximately 5 g

LIGHT HERB AND CHEESE OMELETTE

Preparation time: 5 minutes

Cooking time: 10 minutes

Doses: 1 person

Ingredients:

2 eggs

20 g of light ricotta

30 g of grated cheese

light (parmesan, grana padano)

Fresh chives to taste

Salt and Pepper To Taste

Extra virgin olive oil

(to grease the pan)

Preparation:

In a bowl, beat the eggs with a pinch of salt and pepper. Add the ricotta, grated cheese and chopped chives. Mix the mixture well. Heat a drizzle of oil in a non-stick pan. Pour the egg mixture into the pan and cook the omelette over low heat for about 5 minutes, until the bottom has thickened. Fold the omelette in half and cook for another 23 minutes. Serve hot. You can vary the vegetables and cheese to your liking. For an even lighter version, you can use just egg whites instead of whole eggs.

Nutritional values:

Calories: approximately 250 kcal

Protein: approximately 25 g

Fat: approximately 12 g

Carbohydrates: approximately 3 g

ZUCCHINI TAGLIATELLE
WITH LENTIL SAUCE

Preparation time: 30 minutes

Cooking time: 40 minutes

Doses: 1 person

Ingredients:

1 large courgette

100 g of dried lentils

1/2 small onion

1 small carrot

1 stalk of celery

1 tablespoon of oil

extra virgin olive oil

1 clove of garlic

1 peeled tomato

1 bay leaf

Salt and Pepper To Taste

Fresh basil

chopped (optional)

Preparation:

Wash the lentils and soak them for at least 2 hours. In the meantime, wash the courgette and cut it into thin strips with a potato peeler or a mandolin, creating "tagliatelle". Finely chop the onion, carrot and celery. Heat the oil in a pan. Fry the onion, carrot and celery for a few minutes, until softened. Add the minced garlic and cook for another minute. Add the rinsed lentils, peeled tomato, bay leaf, salt and pepper.

Cover the pot and cook over low heat for about 30 minutes, stirring occasionally, until the lentils are cooked. While the ragù is cooking, cook the courgette "tagliatelle" in boiling salted water for 23 minutes. Drain the courgettes and season them with a drizzle of oil. Serve the courgette "tagliatelle" with the hot lentil ragù, sprinkling with chopped fresh basil (optional).

Nutritional values:

Calories: approximately 400 kcal

Protein: approximately 30 g

Fat: approximately 15 g

Carbohydrates: approximately 10 g

WARM CHICKEN SALAD WITH MUSHROOMS AND SOY

Preparation time: 20 minutes

Cooking time: 15 minutes

Doses: 1 person

Ingredients:

120g sliced chicken breast

100 g of fresh mixed mushrooms

2 tablespoons soy sauce

1 tablespoon of oil

extra virgin olive oil

1/2 small onion

1 clove of garlic

1/2 lemon

Mixed green salad to taste

Sesame seeds (optional)

Preparation:

Wash and slice the mushrooms. Finely chop the onion and garlic. Marinate the chicken with soy sauce, oil, the juice of half a lemon, salt and pepper for at least 15 minutes. Heat the oil in a non-stick pan. Fry the onion and garlic for a few minutes, until softened. Add the mushrooms and cook for 57 minutes, stirring often. Add the marinated chicken and cook it for about 5 minutes on each side, until it is golden and cooked inside.

In the meantime, prepare the salad by washing the lettuce and placing it on a plate. Add the cooked mushrooms and chicken. Season with a drizzle of oil and the juice of half a lemon. Sprinkle with sesame seeds (optional) and serve warm.

Nutritional values:

Calories: approximately 350 kcal

Protein: approximately 40 g

Fat: approximately 12 g

Carbohydrates: approximately 5 g

CONSOLIDATION PHASE

VEGETABLE LASAGNA WITH LIGHT BECHAMEL

Preparation time: 45 minutes

Cooking time: 45 minutes

Doses: 1 person

Ingredients:

2 small aubergines

1 medium courgette

1 red pepper

1 small onion

200 g of light béchamel (prepared

with skimmed milk and wholemeal flour)

50 g of light ricotta

50 g of grated light parmesan

Chopped fresh basil (optional)

Salt and Pepper To Taste

Extra virgin olive oil

(to grease the pan)

Preparation:

Wash the aubergines, courgette and pepper. Cut the aubergines into thin slices lengthwise. Grill the aubergines on both sides for a few minutes, until they are slightly wilted. Cut the courgette and pepper into thin slices. Finely chop the onion. Heat a drizzle of oil in a non-stick pan. Fry the onion for a few minutes, until it softens. Add the courgettes and pepper and cook for 57 minutes, stirring often. In a bowl, mix the light ricotta with the grated parmesan and a pinch of salt and pepper. Prepare the light béchamel following the instructions on the package. Grease a baking tray with oil.

Arrange a layer of grilled aubergines on the bottom of the pan. Spread a little light béchamel on the aubergines. Spread the layer of cooked vegetables (courgettes and peppers). Add a spoonful of the ricotta and parmesan mixture. Repeat the layers until you run out of ingredients. Finish with a layer of light béchamel. Cook in a preheated oven at 180°C for about 30 minutes, until the lasagna is golden and the béchamel sauce is gratinated. Remove from the oven and let rest for a few minutes before serving.

Nutritional values:

Calories: approximately 450 kcal

Protein: approximately 35 g

Fat: approximately 20 g

Carbohydrates: approximately 15 g

CAULIFLOWER AND SHRIMP RISOTTO

Preparation time: 25 minutes

Cooking time: 20 minutes

Doses: 1 person

Ingredients:

150 g of cauliflower

100 g of cleaned shrimps

1/2 small onion

1 clove of garlic

1/2 glass of dry white wine

400 ml of light vegetable broth

1 tablespoon extra virgin olive oil

Chopped fresh parsley

Salt and Pepper To Taste

Preparation:

Wash the cauliflower and cut it into florets. Finely chop the onion and garlic. Fry the onion and garlic in a non-stick pan with oil for a few minutes, until soft. Add the cauliflower florets and cook for 5 minutes, stirring often. Pour in the white wine and let the alcohol evaporate. Add the hot vegetable broth and cook for about 15 minutes, stirring occasionally, until the cauliflower is soft. In the meantime, cook the prawns in another non-stick pan with a drizzle of oil for a couple of minutes on each side, until they are golden.

Add the cooked shrimp to the risotto and mix gently. Season with salt and pepper to taste. Turn off the heat and stir in the risotto with a spoonful of butter (optional). Serve the risotto hot, sprinkled with fresh chopped parsley.

Nutritional values:

Calories: approximately 450 kcal

Protein: approximately 40 g

Fat: approximately 15 g

Carbohydrates: approximately 30 g

PUMPKIN GNOCCHI WITH SOY RAGU

Preparation time: 40 minutes

Cooking time: 30 minutes

Doses: 1 person

Ingredients:

200 g of pumpkin

50 g of wholemeal flour

1 egg

1 tablespoon grated parmesan

Salt and Pepper To Taste

Extra virgin olive oil

(to grease the pan)

For the soy sauce:

100 g of tofu

1/2 small onion

1 clove of garlic

2 tablespoons soy sauce

1 tablespoon extra virgin olive oil

1 peeled tomato

1/2 glass of light vegetable broth

Salt and Pepper To Taste

Preparation:

Wash the pumpkin and cut it into pieces.
Cook the pumpkin by steaming or boiling
water for about 15 minutes, until it is soft.
Mash the pumpkin with a fork to obtain a
puree. Add the wholemeal flour, egg, grated
parmesan, salt and pepper. Knead the
mixture well until you obtain a smooth and
soft dough. If necessary, add a little
wholemeal flour or water to adjust the
consistency. Form gnocchi with wet hands.
Arrange the gnocchi on a floured tray.

For the soy sauce: Crumble the tofu with your hands. Finely chop the onion and garlic. Heat the oil in a non-stick pan. Fry the onion and garlic for a few minutes, until softened. Add the crumbled tofu and cook for 5 minutes, stirring often. Add the soy sauce, peeled tomato, vegetable broth, salt and pepper. Cook the soy sauce for about 15 minutes, stirring occasionally, until it is thick. Add chopped fresh basil (optional). Cooking: Cook the gnocchi in boiling salted water for 23 minutes, until they float to the surface. Drain the gnocchi and season them with the hot soy sauce. Nutritional values:

Calories: approximately 400 kcal

Protein: approximately 35 g

Fat: approximately 15 g

Carbohydrates: approximately 20 g

WHOLE WHOLE PASTA WITH CHICKEN AND MUSHROOMS

Preparation time: 25 minutes

Cooking time: 20 minutes

Doses: 1 person

Ingredients:

80 g of wholemeal pasta

120g sliced chicken breast

100 g of fresh mixed mushrooms

1/2 small onion

1 clove of garlic

1 tablespoon of oil

extra virgin olive oil

1/2 glass of wine

dry white (optional)

Chopped fresh parsley

Salt and Pepper To Taste

Preparation:

Wash and slice the mushrooms. Finely chop the onion and garlic. Marinate the chicken with a pinch of salt and pepper for a few minutes. Heat the oil in a non-stick pan. Fry the onion and garlic for a few minutes, until softened. Add the mushrooms and cook for 57 minutes, stirring often. Add the marinated chicken and cook it for about 5 minutes on each side, until it is golden and cooked inside. Deglaze with dry white wine (optional) and let the alcohol evaporate.

Cook the wholemeal pasta in boiling salted water for the time indicated on the package. Drain the pasta and season it with a drizzle of oil to prevent it from sticking. Add the pasta to the chicken and mushrooms in the pan and mix well. Season with salt and pepper to taste. Serve the pasta hot, sprinkled with chopped fresh parsley.

Nutritional values:

Calories: approximately 400 kcal

Protein: approximately 35 g

Fat: approximately 15 g

Carbohydrates: approximately 25 g

FISH SOUP WITH
PEARL BARLEY

Preparation time: 30 minutes

Cooking time: 40 minutes

Doses: 1 person

Ingredients:

200 g of fresh mixed fish

(cod, sea bream, sea bass)

50 g of pearl barley

1/2 small onion

1 small carrot

1 stalk of celery

1 clove of garlic

1 peeled tomato

1 liter of vegetable broth

1 tablespoon extra virgin olive oil

Chopped fresh parsley

Salt and Pepper To Taste

Preparation:

Wash the fish and cut it into pieces. Wash the pearl barley and soak it for at least 30 minutes. Finely chop the onion, carrot and celery. Fry the onion, carrot and celery in a pan with oil for a few minutes, until soft. Add the minced garlic and cook for another minute. Add the peeled tomato and mash it with a spoon. Add the vegetable broth and bring to the boil.

Add the drained pearl barley and cook for about 20 minutes, until soft. Add the fish and cook for another 10 minutes, until cooked through. Season with salt and pepper to taste. Serve the soup hot, sprinkled with chopped fresh parsley.

Nutritional values:

Calories: approximately 350 kcal

Protein: approximately 30 g

Fat: approximately 10 g

Carbohydrates: approximately 20 g

WHOLE WHOLE CANNELLONI WITH RICOTTA AND BEETS

Preparation time: 40 minutes

Cooking time: 30 minutes

Doses: 1 person

Ingredients:

4 wholemeal cannelloni

200 g of ricotta

150 g of chard

1/2 small onion

1 clove of garlic

1 tablespoon grated parmesan

1 tablespoon extra virgin olive oil

Light béchamel (prepared with milk skimmed and wholemeal flour)

Chopped fresh parsley

Salt and Pepper To Taste

Preparation:

Wash the beets and boil them in boiling salted water for a few minutes. Drain them and squeeze them well. Finely chop the onion and garlic. Fry the onion and garlic in a pan with oil for a few minutes, until soft. Add the chopped beets and cook for 5 minutes, stirring often. In a bowl, mix the ricotta with the grated parmesan, a pinch of salt and pepper. Add the cooked beets and mix well. Cook the wholemeal cannelloni in boiling salted water for the time indicated on the package.

Drain them and fill them with the ricotta and chard mixture. Arrange the cannelloni on a baking tray. Cover the cannelloni with the light béchamel. Cook in a preheated oven at 180°C for about 20 minutes, until the béchamel sauce is gratinated. Remove from the oven and let rest for a few minutes before serving. Sprinkle with chopped fresh parsley.

Nutritional values:

Calories: approximately 400 kcal

Protein: approximately 35 g

Fat: approximately 15 g

Carbohydrates: approximately 25 g

WHOLEWHEAT PIE WITH SEASONAL VEGETABLES

Preparation time: 45 minutes

Cooking time: 40 minutes

Doses: 1 person

Ingredients:

1 roll of wholemeal puff pastry

200 g of seasonal vegetables

(courgettes, peppers, aubergines)

1/2 small onion

1 clove of garlic

1 tablespoon of oil

extra virgin olive oil

2 eggs

50 g of ricotta

50 g of grated parmesan

Chopped fresh parsley

Salt and Pepper To Taste

Preparation:

Wash seasonal vegetables and cut them into small pieces. Finely chop the onion and garlic. Fry the onion and garlic in a pan with oil for a few minutes, until soft. Add the seasonal vegetables and cook them for 1015 minutes, stirring often. In a bowl, beat the eggs with the ricotta, the grated parmesan, a pinch of salt and pepper. Add the cooked vegetables to the egg and ricotta mixture and mix well. Unroll the wholemeal puff pastry and line a baking tray.

Pour the vegetable and ricotta mixture onto the puff pastry. Bake in a preheated oven at 180°C for about 40 minutes, until the savory pie is golden. Remove from the oven and let rest for a few minutes before serving. Sprinkle with chopped fresh parsley.

Nutritional values:

Calories: approximately 450 kcal

Protein: approximately 30 g

Fat: approximately 20 g

Carbohydrates: approximately 30 g

**WHOLE WHOLE PASTA
AND LEGUMES SOUP**

Preparation time: 30 minutes

Cooking time: 40 minutes

Doses: 1 person

Ingredients:

50 g of wholemeal pasta

100 g of mixed legumes

(e.g. chickpeas, lentils, beans)

1/2 small onion

1 small carrot, 1 celery stalk

1 clove of garlic, 1 peeled tomato

1 liter of vegetable broth

1 tablespoon extra virgin olive oil

Chopped fresh parsley

Salt and Pepper To Taste

Preparation:

Rinse the mixed legumes and soak them for at least 30 minutes. Finely chop the onion, carrot and celery. Fry the onion, carrot and celery in a pan with oil for a few minutes, until soft. Add the minced garlic and cook for another minute. Add the peeled tomato and mash it with a spoon. Add the vegetable broth and bring to the boil. Add the drained legumes and cook for about 20 minutes, until they are tender. Add the wholemeal pasta and cook for the time indicated on the package. Season with salt and pepper to taste. Serve the soup hot, sprinkled with fresh chopped parsley. Nutritional values: Calories: approximately 350 kcal

Protein: approximately 30 g, Fat: approximately 10 g

Carbohydrates: approximately 25 g

STABILIZATION PHASE

WHOLE WHOLE PASTA WITH TOMATO AND BASIL

Preparation time: 20 minutes

Cooking time: 20 minutes

Doses: 1 person

Ingredients:

80 g of wholemeal pasta

400 g of peeled tomatoes

1/2 small onion

1 clove of garlic

1 tablespoon extra virgin olive oil

Chopped fresh basil

Salt and Pepper To Taste

Preparation:

Wash the peeled tomatoes and cut them into small pieces. Finely chop the onion and garlic. Fry the onion and garlic in a pan with oil for a few minutes, until soft. Add the peeled tomatoes, a pinch of salt and pepper. Cook for about 15 minutes, stirring occasionally, until the sauce is thick. Cook the wholemeal pasta in boiling salted water for the time indicated on the package. Drain the pasta and season it with the tomato sauce. Add the chopped fresh basil and mix well. Serve the pasta hot.

Nutritional values:

Calories: approximately 350 kcal

Protein: approximately 25 g

Fat: approximately 10 g

Carbohydrates: approximately 30 g

MIXED MUSHROOMS RISOTTO

Preparation time: 25 minutes

Cooking time: 20 minutes

Doses: 1 person

Ingredients:

80 g of Carnaroli rice

100 g of fresh mixed mushrooms

1/2 small onion

1 clove of garlic

1 tablespoon extra virgin olive oil

1/2 glass of dry white wine (optional)

400 ml of light vegetable broth

Chopped fresh parsley

Salt and Pepper To Taste

Preparation:

Wash and slice the mushrooms. Finely chop the onion and garlic. Fry the onion and garlic in a non-stick pan with oil for a few minutes, until soft. Add the mushrooms and cook for 57 minutes, stirring often. Deglaze with dry white wine (optional) and let the alcohol evaporate. Add the Carnaroli rice and toast for a minute. Add the hot vegetable broth one ladle at a time, stirring constantly, and cook for about 15 minutes, until the rice is creamy. Season with salt and pepper to taste. Turn off the heat and stir in the risotto with a spoonful of butter (optional). Serve the risotto hot, sprinkled with fresh chopped parsley. Nutritional values:

Calories: approximately 400 kcal, Proteins: approximately 30 g

Fat: approximately 15 g, Carbohydrates: approximately 25 g

MIXED LEGUME SOUP

Preparation time: 40 minutes

Cooking time: 40 minutes

Doses: 1 person

Ingredients:

100 g of mixed legumes

(chickpeas, lentils, beans)

1/2 small onion

1 small carrot

1 stalk of celery

1 clove of garlic

1 peeled tomato

1 liter of vegetable broth

1 tablespoon extra virgin olive oil

Chopped fresh parsley

Salt and Pepper To Taste

Preparation:

Rinse the mixed legumes and soak them for at least 30 minutes. Finely chop the onion, carrot and celery. Fry the onion, carrot and celery in a pan with oil for a few minutes, until soft. Add the minced garlic and cook for another minute. Add the peeled tomato and mash it with a spoon. Add the vegetable broth and bring to the boil. Add the drained legumes and cook for about 20 minutes, until they are tender. Season with salt and pepper to taste. Serve the soup hot, sprinkled with chopped fresh parsley.

Nutritional values:

Calories: approximately 350 kcal

Protein: approximately 30 g

Fat: approximately 10 g

Carbohydrates: approximately 25 g

WHOLEWHEAT PENNE WITH AUBERGINE DRIED TOMATOES AND BASIL

Preparation time: 30 minutes

Cooking time: 30 minutes

Doses: 1 person

Ingredients:

80 g of wholemeal penne

1 small aubergine

5 dried tomatoes

1/2 small onion

1 clove of garlic

1 tablespoon extra virgin olive oil

Chopped fresh basil

Salt and Pepper To Taste

Preparation:

Wash the aubergine and cut it into cubes. Hydrate the dried tomatoes in warm water for 10 minutes. Finely chop the onion and garlic. Fry the onion and garlic in a pan with oil for a few minutes, until soft. Add the diced aubergine and cook for 10 minutes, stirring often. Add the dried tomatoes, squeezed and cut into pieces. Cook for another 5 minutes, stirring gently. Cook the wholemeal penne in boiling salted water for the time indicated on the package. Drain the pasta and season it with the aubergine and dried tomato sauce. Add the chopped fresh basil and mix well. Serve the penne hot.

Nutritional values:

Calories: approximately 400 kcal, Protein: approximately 25 g

Fat: approximately 15 g, Carbohydrates: approximately 30 g

RICOTTA AND SPINACH GNOCCHI

Preparation time: 30 minutes

Cooking time: 20 minutes

Doses: 1 person

Ingredients:

200 g of ricotta

100 g of spinach

50 g of wholemeal flour

1 egg

1 pinch of nutmeg

Salt and Pepper To Taste

Preparation:

Wash the spinach and boil them in boiling salted water for a minute. Drain them and squeeze them well. In a bowl, mix the ricotta, egg, wholemeal flour, a pinch of nutmeg, salt and pepper. Add the chopped spinach and mix well. Form gnocchi with the mixture obtained. Cook the gnocchi in boiling salted water for a couple of minutes, until they float to the surface. Drain the gnocchi and season them with a drizzle of oil and a pinch of grated parmesan (optional).

Nutritional values:

Calories: approximately 400 kcal

Protein: approximately 35 g

Fat: approximately 15 g

Carbohydrates: approximately 20 g

PENNE WITH GRILLED VEGETABLES AND FETA

Preparation time: 20 minutes

Cooking time: 20 minutes

Doses: 1 person

Ingredients:

80 g of wholemeal Penne

1 small courgette

1 small pepper

1 small aubergine

100 g of feta

1 tablespoon extra virgin olive oil

Chopped fresh basil

Salt and Pepper To Taste

Preparation:

Wash the vegetables and cut them into strips. Grill the vegetables for about 10 minutes, turning them often. Cook the wholemeal penne in boiling salted water for the time indicated on the package. Melt the feta in a pan with a drizzle of oil for a minute. Drain the pasta and season it with the grilled vegetables and melted feta. Add the chopped fresh basil and mix well. Serve the penne hot.

Nutritional values:

Calories: approximately 450 kcal

Protein: approximately 30 g

Fat: approximately 20 g

Carbohydrates: approximately 25 g

WHOLE WHOLE RISOTTO WITH COURGETTES AND PRAWNS

Preparation time: 25 minutes

Cooking time: 20 minutes

Doses: 1 person

Ingredients:

80 g of wholemeal Carnaroli rice

100 g of courgettes

100 g of cleaned shrimps

1/2 small onion

1 clove of garlic

1 tablespoon extra virgin olive oil

1/2 glass of dry white wine (optional)

400 ml of light vegetable broth

Chopped fresh parsley

Salt and Pepper To Taste

Preparation:

Wash the courgettes and cut them into cubes. Shell the prawns and clean them. Finely chop the onion and garlic. Fry the onion and garlic in a non-stick pan with oil for a few minutes, until soft. Add the diced courgettes and cook for 57 minutes, stirring often. Deglaze with dry white wine (optional) and let the alcohol evaporate. Add the wholemeal Carnaroli rice and toast for a minute. Add the hot vegetable broth one ladle at a time, stirring constantly, and cook for about 15 minutes, until the rice is creamy.

Add the shrimp and cook for another 23 minutes. Season with salt and pepper to taste. Turn off the heat and stir in the risotto with a spoonful of butter (optional). Serve the risotto hot, sprinkled with fresh chopped parsley.

Nutritional values:

Calories: approximately 500 kcal

Protein: approximately 40 g

Fat: approximately 20 g

Carbohydrates: approximately 30 g

WHOLE WHOLE TORTELLINI WITH TURKEY SAUCE

Preparation time: 45 minutes

Cooking time: 40 minutes

Doses: 1 person

Ingredients:

200 g of wholemeal tortellini

200 g of minced turkey

1/2 small onion

1 small carrot

1 stalk of celery

1 clove of garlic

400 g of peeled tomatoes

1 tablespoon extra virgin olive oil

Chopped fresh basil

Salt and Pepper To Taste

Preparation:

Finely chop the onion, carrot and celery. Fry the onion, carrot and celery in a pan with oil for a few minutes, until soft. Add the minced garlic and cook for another minute. Add the ground turkey and cook for about 5 minutes, stirring often. Add the peeled tomatoes, a pinch of salt and pepper. Cook for about 20 minutes, stirring occasionally, until the ragù is thick. Cook the wholemeal tortellini in boiling salted water for the time indicated on the package. Drain the tortellini and season them with the turkey ragù. Add the chopped fresh basil and mix well. Serve the tortellini hot. Nutritional values:

Calories: approximately 600 kcal, Proteins: approximately 50 g

Fat: approximately 25 g, Carbohydrates: approximately 40 g

RECIPES
SECOND DISHES

ATTACK PHASE

SALMON FILLET WITH LEMON GRILLED VEGETABLES

Preparation time: 20 minutes

Cooking time: 20 minutes

Doses: 1 person

Ingredients:

150 g of salmon fillet

1 lemon

1 tablespoon extra virgin olive oil

Chopped fresh parsley

Salt and Pepper To Taste

Grilled vegetables to taste

(courgettes, peppers, aubergines)

Preparation:

Wash the salmon fillet and dry it well with kitchen paper. Salt and pepper the salmon on both sides. Squeeze the juice of a lemon onto the salmon and massage gently. Heat the extra virgin olive oil in a non-stick pan. Cook the salmon fillet for about 5 minutes per side, until golden and cooked through. Meanwhile, grill vegetables to taste. Serve the salmon fillet with the grilled vegetables and garnish with chopped fresh parsley.

Nutritional values:

Calories: approximately 450 kcal

Protein: approximately 40 g

Fat: approximately 20 g

Carbohydrates: approximately 5 g

BAKED CHICKEN BREAST WITH AROMATIC HERBS

Preparation time: 20 minutes

Cooking time: 30 minutes

Doses: 1 person

Ingredients:

150 g of chicken breast

1 tablespoon of oil

extra virgin olive oil

1 clove of garlic

Fresh rosemary

Fresh sage

Fresh thyme

Salt and Pepper To Taste

Preparation:

Preheat the oven to 180°C. Wash the chicken breast and dry it well with kitchen paper. In a bowl, mix the extra virgin olive oil, minced garlic, fresh rosemary, fresh sage and fresh thyme. Salt and pepper the chicken breast on both sides. Baste the chicken breast with the herb mixture. Cook the chicken breast in the oven for about 30 minutes, until golden and cooked through. Serve the chicken breast with a side of vegetables of your choice.

Nutritional values:

Calories: approximately 350 kcal

Protein: approximately 45 g

Fat: approximately 15 g

Carbohydrates: approximately 0 g

ASPARAGUS AND MUSHROOM OMELETTES

Preparation time: 15 minutes

Cooking time: 10 minutes

Doses: 1 person

Ingredients:

2 eggs

100 g of asparagus

50 g of mixed mushrooms

1/2 small onion

1 tablespoon of oil

extra virgin olive oil

Chopped fresh parsley

Salt and Pepper To Taste

Preparation:

Wash the asparagus and cut them into small pieces. Wash the mushrooms and cut them into slices. Finely chop the onion. Fry the onion in a non-stick pan with oil for a few minutes, until it softens. Add the asparagus and mushrooms and cook for 5 minutes, stirring often. In a bowl, beat the eggs with a pinch of salt and pepper. Pour the egg mixture into the pan with the asparagus and mushrooms. Cook the omelette for about 5 minutes, until cooked through. Fold the omelette in half and serve. Garnish with chopped fresh parsley.

Nutritional values:

Calories: approximately 300 kcal

Protein: approximately 30 g

Fat: approximately 15 g

Carbohydrates: approximately 5 g

STEAMED SALMON WITH LEMON SAUCE AND HERB

Preparation time: 15 minutes

Cooking time: 10 minutes

Doses: 1 person

Ingredients:

150 g of salmon fillet

1 lemon

1 tablespoon of oil

extra virgin olive oil

Chopped fresh parsley

Chopped fresh dill

Salt and Pepper To Taste

Preparation:

Wash the salmon fillet and dry it well with kitchen paper. Salt and pepper the salmon on both sides. Steam the salmon for about 10 minutes, until cooked. Meanwhile, prepare the lemon and herb sauce: in a bowl, mix the juice of one lemon, the extra virgin olive oil, the chopped fresh parsley and the chopped fresh dill. Serve the steamed salmon with the lemon and herb sauce.

Nutritional values:

Calories: approximately 350 kcal

Protein: approximately 40 g

Fat: approximately 15 g

Carbohydrates: approximately 0 g

GRILLED BEEF FILLET WITH ROASTED TOMATOES

Preparation time: 20 minutes

Cooking time: 20 minutes

Doses: 1 person

Ingredients:

150 g of beef fillet

2 tomatoes

1 tablespoon of oil

extra virgin olive oil

Fresh rosemary

Fresh sage

Salt and Pepper To Taste

Preparation:

Wash the beef fillet and dry it well with kitchen paper. Salt and pepper the beef fillet on both sides. Wash the tomatoes and cut them in half. In a bowl, mix the extra virgin olive oil, fresh rosemary and fresh sage. Brush the tomatoes with the herb mixture. Cook the grilled beef fillet for about 5 minutes on each side, until golden and cooked through. Meanwhile, cook the tomatoes in the oven at 180°C for about 15 minutes, until they are roasted. Serve the beef tenderloin with the roasted tomatoes.

Nutritional values:

Calories: approximately 400 kcal

Protein: approximately 45 g

Fat: approximately 20 g

Carbohydrates: approximately 5 g

GRILLED SWORDFISH WITH SPINACH SIDE DISH

Preparation time: 20 minutes

Cooking time: 15 minutes

Doses: 1 person

Ingredients:

150 g of swordfish

200 g of spinach

1 clove of garlic

1 tablespoon of oil

extra virgin olive oil

Salt and Pepper To Taste

Preparation:

Wash the swordfish and dry it well with kitchen paper. Salt and pepper the swordfish on both sides. Grill the swordfish for about 5 minutes per side, until golden and cooked through. In the meantime, wash the spinach and boil them in boiling salted water for a minute. Drain them and squeeze them well. In a pan, heat the extra virgin olive oil and fry the chopped garlic for a minute. Add the spinach and cook for 5 minutes, stirring often. Serve the swordfish with the sautéed spinach.

Nutritional values:

Calories: approximately 350 kcal

Protein: approximately 40 g

Fat: approximately 15 g

Carbohydrates: approximately 5 g

TUNA SALAD WITH TOMATOES AND CUCUMBERS

Preparation time: 10 minutes

Cooking time: 0

Doses: 1 person

Ingredients:

150g canned tuna

100 g of cherry tomatoes

1 cucumber

1/2 red onion

1 tablespoon of oil

extra virgin olive oil

Chopped fresh parsley

Salt and Pepper To Taste

Preparation:

Wash the cherry tomatoes and cut them in half. Wash the cucumber and cut it into thin slices. Finely chop the red onion. In a bowl, mix the tuna, cherry tomatoes, cucumber, red onion, extra virgin olive oil, chopped fresh parsley, salt and pepper to taste. Serve the fresh tuna salad.

Nutritional values:

Calories: approximately 350 kcal

Protein: approximately 40 g

Fat: approximately 20 g

Carbohydrates: approximately 5 g

**BAKED COD FILLET
WITH TOMATOES
AND OREGANO**

Preparation time: 15 minutes

Cooking time: 20 minutes

Doses: 1 person

Ingredients:

150 g of cod fillet

100 g of cherry tomatoes

1 tablespoon of oil

extra virgin olive oil

Fresh oregano

Salt and Pepper To Taste

Preparation:

Preheat the oven to 180°C. Wash the cod fillet and dry it well with kitchen paper. Salt and pepper the cod fillet on both sides. In a baking pan, grease the bottom with extra virgin olive oil. Arrange the cod fillet in the pan and distribute the cherry tomatoes cut in half. Sprinkle with fresh oregano. Bake in the oven for about 20 minutes, until the cod is cooked. Serve the baked cod fillet with cherry tomatoes and oregano.

Nutritional values:

Calories: approximately 300 kcal

Protein: approximately 45 g

Fat: approximately 10 g

Carbohydrates: approximately 5 g

CRUISE PHASE

CHICKEN CURRY WITH GRILLED VEGETABLES

Preparation time: 25 minutes

Cooking time: 20 minutes

Doses: 1 person

Ingredients:

150 g of chicken breast

1 tablespoon extra virgin olive oil

1 small onion

1 clove of garlic

1 teaspoon curry powder

400ml coconut milk

100 g of grilled vegetables to taste

(courgettes, peppers, aubergines)

Chopped fresh parsley, Salt and pepper to taste

Preparation:

Wash the chicken breast and dry it well with kitchen paper. Cut the chicken breast into cubes. In a non-stick pan, heat the extra virgin olive oil and fry the chopped onion and chopped garlic for a few minutes, until soft. Add the curry powder and mix well. Add the diced chicken breast and cook for 5 minutes, stirring often. Pour in the coconut milk and cook for about 15 minutes, until the chicken is cooked and the sauce has thickened. Add grilled vegetables to taste and mix gently. Serve the chicken curry with chopped fresh parsley.

Nutritional values:

Calories: approximately 500 kcal, Proteins: approximately 45 g

Fat: approximately 25 g, Carbohydrates: approximately 5 g

GRILLED SALMON
WITH CITRUS SAUCE

Preparation time: 15 minutes

Cooking time: 15 minutes

Doses: 1 person

Ingredients:

150 g of salmon fillet

1 lemon

1 orange

1 tablespoon of oil

extra virgin olive oil

Chopped fresh parsley

Salt and Pepper To Taste

Preparation:

Wash the salmon fillet and dry it well with kitchen paper. Salt and pepper the salmon on both sides. Grill the salmon for about 10 minutes per side, until golden and cooked through. In the meantime, prepare the citrus sauce: in a bowl, mix the juice of a lemon, the juice of an orange, the extra virgin olive oil and the chopped fresh parsley. Serve the grilled salmon with the citrus sauce.

Nutritional values:

Calories: approximately 400 kcal

Protein: approximately 40 g

Fat: approximately 20 g

Carbohydrates: approximately 5 g

BEEF STEAK WITH PEPPERS AND ONIONS

Preparation time: 20 minutes

Cooking time: 20 minutes

Doses: 1 person

Ingredients:

150 g of beef steak

1 green pepper

1 small onion

1 tablespoon of oil

extra virgin olive oil

Fresh rosemary

Fresh sage

Salt and Pepper To Taste

Preparation:

Wash the beef steak and dry it well with kitchen paper. Salt and pepper the steak on both sides. Wash the green pepper and cut it into slices. Finely chop the onion. In a non-stick pan, heat the extra virgin olive oil and fry the onion for a few minutes, until it softens. Add the sliced pepper and cook for 5 minutes, stirring often. Grill the steak for about 5 minutes per side, until browned and cooked through. Serve steak with sautéed peppers and onion, garnished with fresh rosemary and fresh sage. Nutritional values:

Calories: approximately 450 kcal

Protein: approximately 50 g

Fat: approximately 20 g

Carbohydrates: approximately 5 g

CHICKEN BREAST STUFFED WITH SPINACH AND SKINNY CHEESE

Preparation time: 25 minutes

Cooking time: 30 minutes

Doses: 1 person

Ingredients:

150 g of chicken breast

200 g of spinach

50 g of ricotta

1 clove of garlic

1 tablespoon of oil

extra virgin olive oil

Fresh sage

Salt and Pepper To Taste

Preparation:

Wash the chicken breast and dry it well with kitchen paper. Open a pocket in the chicken breast with a sharp knife. In a pan, heat the extra virgin olive oil and fry the chopped garlic for a minute. Add the spinach and cook for 5 minutes, stirring often. Drain them and squeeze them well. In a bowl, mix the spinach, ricotta, fresh sage, salt and pepper to taste. Stuff the chicken breast with the spinach and ricotta mixture. Close the chicken breast pocket with cooking string. Cook the chicken breast in the oven at 180°C for about 30 minutes, until golden and cooked. Nutritional values:

Calories: approximately 400 kcal

Protein: approximately 50 g

Fat: approximately 15 g

Carbohydrates: approximately 5 g

GRILLED TUNA WITH SAUCE OF TOMATO AND BASIL

Preparation time: 15 minutes

Cooking time: 10 minutes

Doses: 1 person

Ingredients:

150 g of fresh tuna

200 g of peeled tomatoes

1/2 small onion

1 clove of garlic

1 tablespoon of oil

extra virgin olive oil

Fresh basil

Salt and Pepper To Taste

Preparation:

Wash the fresh tuna and dry it well with kitchen paper. Salt and pepper the tuna on both sides. Grill the tuna for about 5 minutes on each side, until golden and cooked. In the meantime, prepare the tomato and basil sauce: in a pan, heat the extra virgin olive oil and fry the chopped onion and minced garlic for a few minutes, until they soften. Add the peeled tomatoes and mash them with a fork. Cook for about 10 minutes, stirring often, until the sauce has thickened. Add chopped fresh basil, salt and pepper to taste. Serve the grilled tuna with the tomato and basil sauce. Nutritional values:

Calories: approximately 400 kcal

Protein: approximately 50 g

Fat: approximately 15 g

Carbohydrates: approximately 5 g

COD IN PAPER WITH MIXED VEGETABLES

Preparation time: 20 minutes

Cooking time: 20 minutes

Doses: 1 person

Ingredients:

150 g of cod fillet

200 g of mixed vegetables

(courgettes, peppers, carrots)

1/2 small onion

1 clove of garlic

1 tablespoon of oil

extra virgin olive oil

Chopped fresh parsley

Salt and Pepper To Taste

Preparation:

Preheat the oven to 180°C. Wash the cod fillet and dry it well with kitchen paper. Wash the mixed vegetables and cut them into pieces. In a bowl, mix the vegetables with the extra virgin olive oil, salt and pepper to taste. Place the cod fillet on a sheet of baking paper. Distribute the vegetables around the cod. Close the baking paper bag. Bake in the oven for about 20 minutes, until the cod is cooked and the vegetables are soft. Serve the cod in foil with chopped fresh parsley.

Nutritional values:

Calories: approximately 350 kcal

Protein: approximately 45 g

Fat: approximately 10 g

Carbohydrates: approximately 5 g

BAKED TURKEY WITH MEDITERRANEAN SPICES

Preparation time: 25 minutes

Cooking time: 40 minutes

Doses: 1 person

Ingredients:

150g turkey breast

1 tablespoon of oil

extra virgin olive oil

1 teaspoon dried oregano

1/2 teaspoon dried thyme

1/4 teaspoon sweet paprika

Salt and Pepper To Taste

Preparation:

Preheat the oven to 180°C. Wash the turkey breast and dry it well with kitchen paper. In a bowl, mix the extra virgin olive oil, dried oregano, dried thyme, sweet paprika, salt and pepper to taste. Sprinkle the spice mixture over the turkey breast. Place the turkey breast on a baking tray lined with baking paper. Bake in the oven for about 40 minutes, until the turkey is browned and cooked through.

Nutritional values:

Calories: approximately 350 kcal

Protein: approximately 50 g

Fat: approximately 15 g

Carbohydrates: approximately 0 g

VEAL MILANESE WITH MIXED SALAD

Preparation time: 20 minutes

Cooking time: 15 minutes

Doses: 1 person

Ingredients:

150 g of veal slice

1 egg

Durum wheat gluten flour

Bread crumbs

Seed oil for frying

Mixed salad

(lettuce, cherry tomatoes, cucumbers)

Lemon

Extra virgin olive oil

Salt and Pepper To Taste

Preparation:

Beat the egg in a shallow dish. Place the durum wheat gluten flour in another shallow dish. Mix the breadcrumbs with a pinch of salt in a third shallow plate. Dip the veal slice in the durum wheat gluten flour, then in the beaten egg and finally in the breadcrumbs. Heat the vegetable oil in a non-stick pan. Fry the veal slice for about 5 minutes on each side, until golden and cooked. In the meantime, prepare the mixed salad: wash and dry the lettuce, cut the cherry tomatoes and cucumbers. Season the salad with lemon juice, extra virgin olive oil, salt and pepper to taste. Serve the Milanese cutlet with the mixed salad. Nutritional values:

Calories: approximately 500 kcal

Protein: approximately 50 g

Fat: approximately 30 g

Carbohydrates: approximately 5 g

CONSOLIDATION PHASE

OVEN SALMON TROUT WITH POTATOES

Preparation time: 20 minutes

Cooking time: 30 minutes

Doses: 1 person

Ingredients:

150 g of salmon trout

200 g of potatoes

1 tablespoon of oil

extra virgin olive oil

Fresh rosemary

Fresh sage

Salt and Pepper To Taste

Preparation:

Preheat the oven to 180°C. Wash the salmon trout and dry it well with kitchen paper. Salt and pepper the salmon trout on both sides. Peel the potatoes and cut them into slices. Place the sliced potatoes on a baking tray and season them with extra virgin olive oil, salt and pepper to taste. Place the salmon trout on top of the potatoes. Garnish with fresh rosemary and fresh sage. Bake in the oven for about 30 minutes, until the salmon trout is cooked and the potatoes are golden.

Nutritional values:

Calories: approximately 500 kcal

Protein: approximately 40 g

Fat: approximately 25 g

Carbohydrates: approximately 10 g

VEGETABLE ROLLS WITH FETA AND TOMATOES

Preparation time: 20 minutes

Cooking time: 15 minutes

Doses: 1 person

Ingredients:

1 medium courgette

1 medium aubergine

100 g of feta

5 cherry tomatoes

1 tablespoon of oil

extra virgin olive oil

Fresh basil

Salt and Pepper To Taste

Preparation:

Wash the courgette and aubergine and cut them into thin strips. Grill the courgette and aubergine strips for a few minutes on each side, until they are soft. Crumble the feta into a bowl. Cut the cherry tomatoes into small pieces. Mix the feta, cherry tomatoes, extra virgin olive oil, fresh basil, salt and pepper to taste. Place a spoonful of the feta and cherry tomato mixture on each strip of grilled courgette and aubergine. Roll the vegetable strips to form rolls. Serve the vegetable rolls with feta and tomatoes. Nutritional values:

Calories: approximately 350 kcal

Protein: approximately 30 g

Fat: approximately 20 g

Carbohydrates: approximately 5 g

LEMON CHICKEN BREAST WITH BROWN RICE

Preparation time: 20 minutes

Cooking time: 30 minutes

Doses: 1 person

Ingredients:

150 g of chicken breast

1 lemon

1 tablespoon of oil

extra virgin olive oil

Fresh rosemary

Fresh sage

Salt and Pepper To Taste

80 g of brown rice

Preparation:

Wash the chicken breast and dry it well with kitchen paper. Salt and pepper the chicken breast on both sides. In a non-stick pan, heat the extra virgin olive oil and cook the chicken breast for about 5 minutes per side, until golden and cooked. In the meantime, prepare the brown rice: rinse the rice under running water and cook it in boiling salted water for about 30 minutes, until it is soft. Serve the lemon chicken breast with brown rice, garnished with fresh rosemary and fresh sage.

Nutritional values:

Calories: approximately 450 kcal

Protein: approximately 50 g

Fat: approximately 15 g

Carbohydrates: approximately 20 g

TURKEY SCALLOPPINE WITH MUSHROOMS AND PARSLEY

Preparation time: 25 minutes

Cooking time: 20 minutes

Doses: 1 person

Ingredients:

150 g of turkey slices

200 g of mixed mushrooms

1/2 small onion

1 clove of garlic

1 tablespoon of oil

extra virgin olive oil

Chopped fresh parsley

Salt and Pepper To Taste

Preparation:

Wash the turkey slices and dry them well with kitchen paper. Salt and pepper the turkey slices on both sides. In a non-stick pan, heat the extra virgin olive oil and fry the chopped onion and chopped garlic for a few minutes, until soft. Add the mixed mushrooms and cook them for about 5 minutes, stirring often. Add the turkey slices and cook them for about 5 minutes on each side, until they are golden and cooked. Add the chopped fresh parsley and mix gently. Serve the turkey escalopes with mushrooms and parsley. Nutritional values:

Calories: approximately 400 kcal

Protein: approximately 45 g

Fat: approximately 15 g

Carbohydrates: approximately 5 g

SALMON IN PAPER WITH VEGETABLES AND PESTO

Preparation time: 20 minutes

Cooking time: 20 minutes

Doses: 1 person

Ingredients:

150 g of salmon fillet

200 g of mixed vegetables (for example, courgettes, peppers, carrots)

1 tablespoon pesto

1/2 small onion

1 clove of garlic

1 tablespoon extra virgin olive oil

Chopped fresh parsley

Salt and Pepper To Taste

Preparation:

Preheat the oven to 180°C. Wash the salmon fillet and dry it well with kitchen paper. Wash the mixed vegetables and cut them into pieces. In a bowl, mix the vegetables with the extra virgin olive oil, salt and pepper to taste. Place the salmon fillet on a sheet of baking paper. Arrange the vegetables around the salmon. Add the pesto and chopped fresh parsley. Close the baking paper bag. Bake in the oven for about 20 minutes, until the salmon is cooked and the vegetables are soft.

Nutritional values:

Calories: approximately 450 kcal

Protein: approximately 45 g

Fat: approximately 20 g

Carbohydrates: approximately 5 g

CHICKPEA AND LENTIL VEGETARIAN BURGER

Preparation time: 30 minutes

Cooking time: 20 minutes

Doses: 1 person

Ingredients:

100 g of dried chickpeas

100 g of dried lentils

1 small onion

1 clove of garlic

1 carrot

1 stalk of celery

1 tablespoon breadcrumbs

1/2 teaspoon cumin

1/4 teaspoon sweet paprika

1/4 teaspoon turmeric

Salt and Pepper To Taste

Extra virgin olive oil for frying

Preparation:

Rinse the chickpeas and lentils under running water and soak them for at least 12 hours. Drain them and rinse them again. In a saucepan, cook the chickpeas and lentils in boiling water for about 30 minutes, until soft. Meanwhile, chop the onion, garlic, carrot and celery. In a non-stick pan, heat a drizzle of extra virgin olive oil and fry the chopped vegetables for a few minutes, until wilted. Drain the cooked chickpeas and lentils and mash them with a fork.

Combine the chopped vegetables, breadcrumbs, cumin, sweet paprika, turmeric, salt and pepper to taste. Mix the mixture well and form two burgers. In a non-stick pan, heat a drizzle of extra virgin olive oil and cook the vegetarian burgers for about 5 minutes per side, until they are golden and cooked.

Nutritional values:

Calories: approximately 400 kcal

Protein: approximately 30 g

Fat: approximately 15 g

Carbohydrates: approximately 20 g

GRILLED BEEF FILLET WITH GRILLED VEGETABLES

Preparation time: 20 minutes

Cooking time: 15 minutes

Doses: 1 person

Ingredients:

150 g of beef fillet

200 g of mixed vegetables (for example, courgettes, peppers, aubergines)

1 tablespoon extra virgin olive oil

Fresh rosemary

Fresh sage

Salt and Pepper To Taste

Preparation:

Wash the beef fillet and dry it well with kitchen paper. Salt and pepper the beef fillet on both sides. Wash the mixed vegetables and cut them into pieces. In a non-stick pan, heat the extra virgin olive oil and grill the vegetables for a few minutes on each side, until they are soft. Grill the beef fillet for about 5 minutes per side, until browned and cooked through. Serve the grilled beef fillet with the grilled vegetables, garnished with fresh rosemary and fresh sage.

Nutritional values:

Calories: approximately 450 kcal

Protein: approximately 50 g

Fat: approximately 20 g

Carbohydrates: approximately 5 g

VEGETABLE OMELETTE WITH LIGHT CHEESE

Preparation time: 20 minutes

Cooking time: 10 minutes

Doses: 1 person

Ingredients:

2 eggs

200 g of mixed vegetables (for example, courgettes, peppers, onions)

50 g of grated light cheese

1 tablespoon extra virgin olive oil

Fresh basil

Salt and Pepper To Taste

Preparation:

Beat the eggs in a bowl with a pinch of salt. Wash the mixed vegetables and cut them into small pieces. In a non-stick pan, heat the extra virgin olive oil and fry the vegetables for a few minutes, until they are wilted. Pour the beaten eggs into the pan and mix gently. Add the grated light cheese and the chopped fresh basil. Cook the omelette for about 5 minutes, until cooked. Fold the omelette in half and serve hot.

Nutritional values:

Calories: approximately 350 kcal

Protein: approximately 30 g

Fat: approximately 15 g

Carbohydrates: approximately 5 g

STABILIZATION PHASE

SEABASS IN SALT WITH SEASONAL VEGETABLES

Preparation time: 30 minutes

Cooking time: 45 minutes

Doses: 1 person

Ingredients:

1 whole sea bass weighing approximately 500 g

1 kg of coarse salt

200 g of seasonal vegetables (for example, tomatoes, courgettes, potatoes)

1 tablespoon extra virgin olive oil

Chopped fresh parsley

Salt and Pepper To Taste

Preparation:

Preheat the oven to 200°C. Wash the sea bass and dry it well with kitchen paper. In a baking pan, place a layer of coarse salt. Place the sea bass on the bed of salt. Distribute the seasonal vegetables around the sea bass. Cover the sea bass with another layer of coarse salt, sealing the edges well. Bake in the oven for about 45 minutes. Remove the pan from the oven and leave to rest for a few minutes. Break the salt crust with a spoon and remove the sea bass. Remove the skin and fins of the sea bass. Flake the sea bass meat with a fork. Season the sea bass with a drizzle of extra virgin olive oil, chopped fresh parsley, salt and pepper to taste. Serve the salted sea bass with seasonal vegetables. Nutritional values:

Calories: approximately 500 kcal, Proteins: approximately 60 g

Fat: approximately 15 g, Carbohydrates: approximately 5 g

CHICKEN SCALOPPINE WITH MUSHROOMS AND MASHED POTATOES

Preparation time: 30 minutes

Cooking time: 20 minutes

Doses: 1 person

Ingredients:

150 g of chicken breast slices

200 g of mixed mushrooms

1/2 small onion

1 clove of garlic

1 tablespoon extra virgin olive oil

Chopped fresh parsley

Salt and Pepper To Taste

200 g of potatoes

Skimmed milk to taste

Preparation:

Wash the chicken breast slices and dry them well with kitchen paper. Salt and pepper the chicken breast slices on both sides. In a non-stick pan, heat the extra virgin olive oil and fry the chopped onion and chopped garlic for a few minutes, until soft. Add the mixed mushrooms and cook them for about 5 minutes, stirring often. Add the chicken breast slices and cook them for about 5 minutes per side, until they are golden and cooked. Meanwhile, prepare the mashed potatoes: peel the potatoes and cut them into pieces.

Cook the potatoes in boiling salted water for about 15 minutes, until they are soft. Mash the potatoes with a fork and add a little skimmed milk to obtain a creamy mixture. Serve the chicken cutlets with mushrooms with the mashed potatoes, garnished with chopped fresh parsley. Nutritional values:

Calories: approximately 550 kcal

Protein: approximately 50 g

Fat: approximately 20 g

Carbohydrates: approximately 30 g

TURKEY BURGER WITH WHEEL BREAD AND GRILLED VEGETABLES

Preparation time: 25 minutes

Cooking time: 20 minutes

Doses: 1 person

Ingredients:

150 g of minced turkey

1 wholemeal sandwich

1/2 small onion

1 tomato

1 courgette

1 aubergine

1 tablespoon extra virgin olive oil

Chopped fresh parsley

Salt and Pepper To Taste

Preparation:

Wash the courgette and aubergine and cut them into slices. Grill the courgette and aubergine slices for a few minutes on each side, until they are soft. In a non-stick pan, heat the extra virgin olive oil and fry the chopped onion for a few minutes, until it softens. Add the ground turkey and cook it by crumbling it with a wooden spoon for about 5 minutes, until it is browned. Salt and pepper the turkey mixture. Heat the wholemeal sandwich. Assemble the hamburger: spread a little chopped fresh parsley on the wholemeal bun, add the turkey mixture, the tomato slices and the grilled courgette and aubergine slices. Close the sandwich and serve the turkey burger with grilled vegetables. Nutritional values:

Calories: approximately 450 kcal, Protein: approximately 40 g

Fat: approximately 15 g, Carbohydrates: approximately 20 g

SALMON FILLET PISTACHIO CRUST WITH WHOLE WHOLE COUS COUS

Preparation time: 30 minutes

Cooking time: 25 minutes

Doses: 1 person

Ingredients:

150 g of salmon fillet

50 g of chopped pistachios

2 tablespoons of breadcrumbs

1 tablespoon extra virgin olive oil

Chopped fresh parsley

Salt and Pepper To Taste

80 g of wholemeal couscous

Vegetable broth to taste

Preparation:

Preheat the oven to 200°C.

Wash the salmon fillet and dry it well with kitchen paper. In a bowl, mix the chopped pistachios, breadcrumbs, extra virgin olive oil, chopped fresh parsley, salt and pepper to taste. Spread the pistachio mixture over the salmon fillet. Arrange the pistachio crusted salmon fillet on a baking tray lined with baking paper. Bake in the oven for about 20 minutes, until the salmon is cooked and the crust is golden. In the meantime, prepare the wholemeal couscous: in a pan, bring the vegetable broth to the boil. Remove from the heat and add the wholemeal couscous. Cover the pan with a cloth and leave to rest for about 5 minutes. Fluff the whole couscous with a fork. Serve the salmon fillet in a pistachio crust with the wholemeal couscous. Nutritional values:

Calories: approximately 500 kcal, Proteins: approximately 45 g

Fat: approximately 20 g, Carbohydrates: approximately 30 g

BEEF STEAK WITH GRILLED PEPPERS

Preparation time: 20 minutes

Cooking time: 20 minutes

Doses: 1 person

Ingredients:

150 g of beef steak

2 peppers

1 tablespoon of oil

extra virgin olive oil

Fresh rosemary

Fresh sage

Salt and Pepper To Taste

Preparation:

Wash the beef steak and dry it well with kitchen paper. Salt and pepper the beef steak on both sides. Wash the peppers and cut them into slices. Grill the sirloin steak for about 5 minutes per side, until cooked through. Grill the peppers for about 10 minutes, until soft. Serve the sirloin steak with the grilled peppers, garnished with fresh rosemary and fresh sage.

Nutritional values:

Calories: approximately 450 kcal

Protein: approximately 50 g

Fat: approximately 20 g

Carbohydrates: approximately 5 g

AUBERGINE ROLLS WITH VEGETABLES AND LIGHT CHEESE

Preparation time: 30 minutes

Cooking time: 20 minutes

Doses: 1 person

Ingredients:

1 aubergine

100 g of courgettes

50 g of grated light cheese

1 tablespoon of oil

extra virgin olive oil

Fresh basil

Salt and Pepper To Taste

Preparation:

Wash the aubergine and cut it into thin slices. Grill the aubergine slices for a few minutes on each side, until they are softened. Wash the courgettes and cut them into strips. In a non-stick pan, heat the extra virgin olive oil and fry the courgettes for a few minutes, until they are soft. Add the grated light cheese and the chopped fresh basil, mixing well. Place a spoonful of the zucchini and cheese mixture on each slice of grilled aubergine. Roll the aubergine slices to form rolls. Serve the aubergine rolls with vegetables and light cheese. Nutritional values:

Calories: approximately 350 kcal, Protein: approximately 30 g

Fat: approximately 15 g, Carbohydrates: approximately 5 g

SLICED BEEF WITH MIXED SALAD AND SEASONED TOMATOES

Preparation time: 20 minutes

Cooking time: 15 minutes

Doses: 1 person

Ingredients:

200 g of cut beef

100 g of mixed salad

(lettuce, rocket, valerian)

10 cherry tomatoes

1 tablespoon extra virgin olive oil

Balsamic vinegar to taste

Salt and Pepper To Taste

Preparation:

Grill the steak for about 5 minutes per side, until cooked to your liking. Wash the mixed salad and cut it into pieces. Wash the cherry tomatoes and cut them in half. In a bowl, season the mixed salad with extra virgin olive oil, balsamic vinegar, salt and pepper to taste. Arrange the mixed salad on a serving plate. Slice the beef steak and arrange it over the salad. Decorate with the seasoned cherry tomatoes.

Nutritional values:

Calories: approximately 500 kcal

Protein: approximately 60 g

Fat: approximately 20 g

Carbohydrates: approximately 5 g

SWORDFISH WITH LEMON WITH BULGUR AND VEGETABLES

Preparation time: 30 minutes

Cooking time: 20 minutes

Doses: 1 person

Ingredients:

200 g of swordfish

80 g of bulgur

100 g of mixed vegetables (for example, courgettes, peppers, onions)

1 tablespoon extra virgin olive oil

Juice of 1 lemon

Chopped fresh parsley

Salt and Pepper To Taste

Preparation:

Cook the bulgur in boiling salted water for about 15 minutes, until soft. Wash the swordfish and cut it into slices. Wash the mixed vegetables and cut them into small pieces. In a non-stick pan, heat the extra virgin olive oil and fry the vegetables for a few minutes, until they are wilted. Add the swordfish steaks and cook them for about 5 minutes on each side, until they are cooked. Add the lemon juice and cook for another minute. Drain the bulgur and add it to the vegetables and swordfish. Season with chopped fresh parsley, salt and pepper to taste. Nutritional values:

Calories: approximately 450 kcal

Protein: approximately 50 g

Fat: approximately 15 g

Carbohydrates: approximately 20 g

SIDE DISH RECIPES

ATTACK PHASE

CUCUMBER AND TOMATO SALAD WITH APPLE VINEGAR AND AROMATIC HERBS

Preparation time: 15 minutes

Cooking time:

Doses: 1 person

Ingredients:

1 medium cucumber

1 medium tomato

1 tablespoon extra virgin olive oil

1 tablespoon apple cider vinegar

1/2 teaspoon dried oregano

1/4 teaspoon dried thyme

Salt and Pepper To Taste

Preparation:

Wash the cucumber and tomato. Cut the cucumber into thin slices and the tomato into cubes. In a bowl, mix the cucumber, tomato, extra virgin olive oil, apple cider vinegar, dried oregano, dried thyme, salt and pepper to taste. Serve the fresh cucumber and tomato salad.

Nutritional values:

Calories: approximately 150 kcal

Protein: approximately 2 g

Fat: approximately 10 g

Carbohydrates: approximately 5 g

GRILLED ASPARAGUS WITH OLIVE OIL AND BLACK PEPPER

Preparation time: 10 minutes

Cooking time: 10 minutes

Doses: 1 person

Ingredients:

150 g of asparagus

1 tablespoon of oil

extra virgin olive oil

Black pepper to taste

Preparation:

Wash the asparagus and cut the tough end part. Grill the asparagus for about 10 minutes, turning often, until tender. Season the grilled asparagus with extra virgin olive oil and black pepper to taste. Serve the grilled asparagus hot.

Nutritional values:

Calories: approximately 100 kcal

Protein: approximately 3 g

Fat: approximately 8 g

Carbohydrates: approximately 3 g

SAUTÉED CHAMPIGNON MUSHROOMS WITH GARLIC AND PARSLEY

Preparation time: 15 minutes

Cooking time: 10 minutes

Doses: 1 person

Ingredients:

200 g of champignon mushrooms

1 clove of garlic

1 tablespoon of oil

extra virgin olive oil

Chopped fresh parsley

Salt and Pepper To Taste

Preparation:

Wash the champignon mushrooms and cut them into slices. In a non-stick pan, heat the extra virgin olive oil and fry the chopped garlic for a minute. Add the button mushrooms and cook for about 10 minutes, stirring often, until they are tender. Season the sautéed champignon mushrooms with chopped fresh parsley, salt and pepper to taste. Serve the sautéed champignon mushrooms hot.

Nutritional values:

Calories: approximately 150 kcal

Protein: approximately 3 g

Fat: approximately 10 g

Carbohydrates: approximately 5 g

CRUISE PHASE

GRILLED COURGETTES WITH PEPPERS AND ONIONS

Preparation time: 20 minutes

Cooking time: 20 minutes

Doses: 1 person

Ingredients:

1 medium courgette

1/2 bell pepper

1/2 onion

1 tablespoon of oil

extra virgin olive oil

Dried oregano to taste

Salt and Pepper To Taste

Preparation:

Wash the courgette, pepper and onion. Cut the courgette into slices, the pepper into strips and the onion into rings. Grill the vegetables for about 10 minutes per side, until soft. Season the grilled vegetables with extra virgin olive oil, dried oregano, salt and pepper to taste. Serve the grilled vegetables hot.

Nutritional values:

Calories: approximately 150 kcal

Protein: approximately 2 g

Fat: approximately 10 g

Carbohydrates: approximately 5 g

BAKED AUBERGINES WITH TOMATO AND BASIL SAUCE

Preparation time: 30 minutes

Cooking time: 30 minutes

Doses: 1 person

Ingredients:

1 medium aubergine

200 g of tomato sauce

Fresh basil

Extra virgin olive oil to taste

Salt and Pepper To Taste

Preparation:

Preheat the oven to 180°C. Wash the aubergine and cut it into slices. Arrange the aubergine slices on a baking tray lined with baking paper. Season the aubergines with extra virgin olive oil, salt and pepper to taste. Pour the tomato sauce over the aubergines. Bake in the oven for about 30 minutes, until the aubergines are soft. Garnish with fresh basil leaves. Serve the baked aubergines with hot tomato and basil sauce.

Nutritional values:

Calories: approximately 250 kcal

Protein: approximately 8 g

Fat: approximately 15 g

Carbohydrates: approximately 10 g

MIXED SALAD WITH CHICORY, LETTUCE, ARUGULA AND GRATED CARROTS

Preparation time: 10 minutes

Cooking time:

Doses: 1 person

Ingredients:

50 g of chicory

50 g of lettuce

30 g of arugula

1 medium carrot

1 tablespoon of oil

extra virgin olive oil

Lemon juice to taste

Salt and Pepper To Taste

Preparation:

Wash the radicchio, lettuce and rocket. Cut the radicchio into strips and the lettuce into leaves. Grate the carrot. In a bowl, mix the radicchio, lettuce, rocket, grated carrot, extra virgin olive oil, lemon juice, salt and pepper to taste. You can add other vegetables of your choice to the grilled vegetables, such as tomatoes or mushrooms.

Serve the fresh mixed salad.

Nutritional values:

Calories: approximately 100 kcal

Protein: approximately 3 g

Fat: approximately 5 g

Carbohydrates: approximately 5 g

CONSOLIDATION PHASE

COLD QUINOA WITH PEPPERS, TOMATOES AND BLACK OLIVES

Preparation time: 20 minutes

Cooking time: 15 minutes

Doses: 1 person

Ingredients:

80 g of quinoa

1/2 bell pepper

10 cherry tomatoes

10 black olives

1 tablespoon of oil

extra virgin olive oil

Dried oregano to taste

Salt and Pepper To Taste

Preparation:

Cook the quinoa in boiling salted water for about 15 minutes, until cooked. Wash the pepper and cut it into small pieces. Wash the cherry tomatoes and cut them in half. Drain the quinoa and season it with extra virgin olive oil, salt and pepper to taste. Add the bell pepper, cherry tomatoes and black olives to the quinoa. Mix well and leave to rest in the refrigerator for at least 30 minutes before serving.

Nutritional values:

Calories: approximately 350 kcal

Protein: approximately 15 g

Fat: approximately 15 g

Carbohydrates: approximately 30 g

BAKED SWEET POTATOES WITH ROSEMARY AND GARLIC

Preparation time: 15 minutes

Cooking time: 45 minutes

Doses: 1 person

Ingredients:

1 medium sweet potato

1 clove of garlic

1 sprig of rosemary

1 tablespoon of oil

extra virgin olive oil

Salt and Pepper To Taste

Preparation:

Preheat the oven to 200°C. Wash the sweet potato and peel it. Cut the sweet potato into slices about 1cm thick. Arrange the sweet potato slices on a baking tray lined with baking paper. Season the sweet potatoes with extra virgin olive oil, salt and pepper to taste. Add the chopped garlic and the rosemary sprig. Bake for about 45 minutes, until the sweet potatoes are soft.

Nutritional values:

Calories: approximately 200 kcal

Protein: approximately 2 g

Fat: approximately 10 g

Carbohydrates: approximately 30 g

COURGETTE FLAN WITH RICOTTA AND EGGS

Preparation time: 20 minutes

Cooking time: 30 minutes

Doses: 1 person

Ingredients:

200 g of courgettes

100 g of ricotta

2 eggs

2 tablespoons of

grated Parmesan cheese

Salt and Pepper To Taste

Preparation:

Wash the courgettes and grate them. In a bowl, mix the grated courgettes, ricotta, eggs, grated parmesan, salt and pepper to taste. Pour the mixture onto a baking tray lined with baking paper. Bake in the oven at 180°C for about 30 minutes, until the flan is golden. You can add other ingredients of your choice to the cold quinoa, such as feta, corn or chickpeas. You can use another type of herb for baked sweet potatoes, such as thyme or sage. If you prefer, you can cook the courgette flan in a pan over low heat for about 20 minutes. Nutritional values:

Calories: approximately 250 kcal

Protein: approximately 20 g

Fat: approximately 15 g

Carbohydrates: approximately 5 g

STABILIZATION PHASE

WHOLE WHOLE COUSCOUS WITH GRILLED VEGETABLES AND FRESH MINT

Preparation time: 20 minutes

Cooking time: 10 minutes

Doses: 1 person

Ingredients:

80 g of wholemeal couscous

1 medium courgette

1/2 bell pepper

1 red onion

1 tablespoon of oil

extra virgin olive oil

Fresh mint to taste

Salt and Pepper To Taste

Preparation:

Cook the wholemeal couscous in boiling salted water for about 10 minutes, until cooked. Wash the courgette, pepper and red onion. Cut the courgette into slices, the pepper into strips and the onion into rings. Grill the vegetables for about 10 minutes per side, until soft. Drain the wholemeal couscous and season it with extra virgin olive oil, salt and pepper to taste. Add the grilled vegetables to the couscous and mix well. Garnish with fresh mint leaves. Serve wholemeal couscous with grilled vegetables and warm fresh mint.

Nutritional values:

Calories: approximately 350 kcal

Protein: approximately 15 g

Fat: approximately 15 g

Carbohydrates: approximately 30 g

BAKED POTATOES WITH ROSEMARY AND GARLIC

Preparation time: 15 minutes

Cooking time: 45 minutes

Doses: 1 person

Ingredients:

1 medium potato

1 clove of garlic

1 sprig of rosemary

1 tablespoon of oil

extra virgin olive oil

Salt and Pepper To Taste

Preparation:

Preheat the oven to 200°C. Wash the potato and peel it. Cut the potato into slices about 1 cm thick. Arrange the potato slices on a baking tray lined with baking paper. Season the potatoes with extra virgin olive oil, salt and pepper to taste. Add the chopped garlic and the rosemary sprig. Bake in the oven for about 45 minutes, until the potatoes are soft.

Nutritional values:

Calories: approximately 200 kcal

Protein: approximately 2 g

Fat: approximately 10 g

Carbohydrates: approximately 30 g

MIXED VEGETABLE OMELETTE WITH SPINACH, TOMATOES AND COURGETTES

Preparation time: 20 minutes

Cooking time: 15 minutes

Doses: 1 person

Ingredients:

2 eggs

50 g of spinach

5 cherry tomatoes

1/2 courgette

1 tablespoon of oil

extra virgin olive oil

Salt and Pepper To Taste

Preparation:

Wash the spinach, cherry tomatoes and courgette. Fry the chopped courgette in a non-stick pan with a spoonful of extra virgin olive oil for a couple of minutes. Add the spinach and cook for another minute, until wilted. Add the cherry tomatoes cut in half and cook for a minute. In a bowl, beat the eggs with a pinch of salt and pepper. Pour the egg mixture into the pan with the vegetables and cook over low heat for about 10 minutes, until the omelette is cooked. Fold the omelette in half and serve hot.

Nutritional values:

Calories: approximately 250 kcal

Protein: approximately 20 g

Fat: approximately 15 g

Carbohydrates: approximately 5 g

CONCLUSION

As we conclude our journey together through the Dukan Diet 2024, I sincerely hope that you have found inspiration, motivation, and most importantly, tangible results on your journey to wellness and your desired weight. I kindly invite you to share your experience and feedback about this book. Reviews are critical to helping other readers discover the value of this program and to supporting the author's work. If you enjoyed the book and it had a positive impact on your life, I would be extremely grateful if you could take a few minutes of your time to leave a review. Your opinion matters and can make a difference to those looking for reliable guidance in their quest for health and wellness.

Thank you for dedicating your time and attention to these pages, for showing a sincere interest in understanding and improving your health. Your words could be a guiding light for other wellness seekers embarking on this path. I thank you deeply for choosing The Dukan Diet 2024. Thank you very much for choosing to accompany me on this journey and for investing in your health and well-being. I wish you all the success and happiness in your future journey.With gratitude, **TERY LONG**